Getting the
Message Across

GETTING THE MESSAGE ACROSS

COMMUNICATION WITH DIVERSE POPULATIONS IN CLINICAL GENETICS

Edited by
Jennifer Wiggins
and
Anna Middleton

OXFORD
UNIVERSITY PRESS

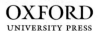

Oxford University Press is a department of the University of Oxford.
It furthers the University's objective of excellence in research, scholarship,
and education by publishing worldwide.

Oxford   New York
Auckland   Cape Town   Dar es Salaam   Hong Kong   Karachi
Kuala Lumpur   Madrid   Melbourne   Mexico City   Nairobi
New Delhi   Shanghai   Taipei   Toronto

With offices in
Argentina   Austria   Brazil   Chile   Czech Republic   France   Greece
Guatemala   Hungary   Italy   Japan   Poland   Portugal   Singapore
South Korea   Switzerland   Thailand   Turkey   Ukraine   Vietnam

Oxford is a registered trademark of Oxford University Press in the UK and certain other
countries.

Published in the United States of America by
Oxford University Press
198 Madison Avenue, New York, NY 10016

© Oxford University Press 2013

Library of Congress Cataloging-in-Publication Data
Getting the message across : communication with diverse populations in clinical genetics /
edited by Jennifer Wiggins, Anna Middleton.
    p. ; cm.
Includes bibliographical references and index.
ISBN 978–0–19–975741–1 (pbk. : alk. paper)—ISBN 978–0–19–997737–6 (e-book)
I. Wiggins, Jennifer.   II. Middleton, Anna.
[DNLM: 1. Genetic Counseling—methods—Great Britain.   2. Communication
Barriers—Great Britain.   3. Cultural Diversity—Great Britain.   4. Disabled Persons—Great
Britain. QZ 50]
616'.042—dc23
2012032187

9 8 7 6 5 4 3 2 1
Printed in the United States of America
on acid-free paper

Contents

Foreword

Communication is a fundamental element of genetic counseling practice and requires particular skill because the information being conveyed by the professional is often both complex as well as laden with potential personal and familial significance for the client/patient and his or her family. When the genetic counselor is also faced with patients who, for sensory, cognitive, linguistic, or cultural reasons, present potential barriers, communication becomes an even greater challenge. Additional skills are also needed for particularly sensitive situations including consultations with the parents of newborns with indeterminate sex or those individuals as adults, the disclosure by patients of sexual abuse, or when discussing genetic testing with terminally ill patients. All too often, because of time and other resource pressures, or lack of preparation, as genetic counselors we are left with feeling that the consultation was less than satisfactory, that we have let these clients down. Although we may need to live with some of the institutional/structural limitations of the service we can provide, we have a professional responsibility to ensure that our practice is not poorer through lack of awareness or skill. For the first time, the editors of this welcome new text have consolidated specialist expertise so that we can work toward improving the quality of our communication with these specific client groups.

Each of the contributing authors give substantial background information, including research evidence where available, goes on to set this in the context of genetic counseling cases, and, perhaps most helpfully, gives very many specific suggestions for practice that range from practical arrangements in the clinic to the actual words that might be used to frame a particular intervention. In my own view, written accounts of counseling skills can often be too vague and generic, lacking clear detail. All of the chapters in this book avoid that pitfall, the topics being presented really come alive, and the pages are full to the brim with imaginative and helpful tips for practice.

I hope that this book enjoys the wide readership it deserves. Both genetic counselors and medical geneticists, whether in training or with years of experience, will find much to learn here, as I have done when privileged to be among the first readers. Many will want to read through the text in its entirety. Some sections, such as the chapters on talking to teenagers, working with particular cultural groups, and using interpreters, will be a great addition to the reading lists for postgraduate genetic counseling training programmes. Trainee and experienced medical geneticists should find the chapters on talking to children and parents with learning difficulties, and parents of newborns with indeterminate sex very relevant. Individual chapters will also become useful for experienced clinical genetic professionals to refer to when seeing a client with communication needs not usually encountered in their practice, for example a deaf patient in a cancer genetic clinic, or a genetic counselor receiving the disclosure of sexual abuse in a consultation for the first time.

On a personal note, I am delighted to see the publication of this book, which indicates a further maturation of our profession. It is to the great credit of the two genetic counselor-editors that they have brought together contributions from a diverse group of experts (many of whom are genetic counselors themselves) to produce a text that contains thoughtful and in-depth coverage around many of the most challenging and complex counseling situations encountered in genetic practice.

Prof Lauren Kerzin-Storrar

Consultant Genetic Counselor (Head) and MSc Course Director

Genetic Medicine

Manchester Academic Health Sciences Centre/CMFT

St Mary's Hospital, Manchester, United Kingdom

Definition of Genetic Counseling

Genetic counseling is the process of helping people understand and adapt to the medical, psychological, and familial implications of genetic contribution to disease. This process integrates the following:

- Interpretation of family and medical histories to assess the chance of disease occurrence or recurrence
- Education about inheritance, testing, management, prevention, resources, and research
- Counseling to promote informed choices and adaptation to risk or condition
  Definition from the National Society of Genetic Counselors (Resta 2006)

SCOPE OF PRACTICE OF GENETIC COUNSELORS

- Collect and interpret comprehensive client information, including medical, psychological, and genetic family history
- Make appropriate and accurate genetic risk assessments
- Use therapeutic counseling and communication skills with clients to help them:
  - comprehend medical facts about a genetic disorder
  - appreciate the way heredity contributes to the disorder, and the risk of recurrence in specific relatives
  - understand options for dealing with the risk of recurrence
  - choose the course of action that seems to them appropriate
  - make the best possible adjustment to the disorder in an affected family member and/or the risk of recurrence of that disorder
- Make psychosocial assessments of client need, providing support and referral to other agencies as appropriate
- Plan, organize, and deliver professional and public education in genetic healthcare
- Serve as a genetic healthcare resource for professionals and the general public
- Liaise with other members of the genetics multidisciplinary team to provide optimum services for clients
  Genetic Counselor Registration Board UK and ROI Code of Conduct (2012)

Preface

The two words "information" and "communication" are often used interchangeably, but they signify quite different things. Information is giving out; communication is getting through.

—Sidney J Harris

The idea for this book developed from a plenary session at the British Society of Human Genetics annual conference in 2008. This session was called "Getting the Message Across: Communication Challenges in Clinical Genetics." It had been organized by senior genetic counselors Jennifer Wiggins and Vicki Wiles on behalf of the Association of Genetic Counselors and Nurses (U.K.), and Dr. Anna Middleton was one of the presenters. There appeared to be a demand from the audience for practical tips that support cross-cultural genetic counseling. We wanted to build on the session by creating this book and invited genetic counselors with a particular expertise developed through research interests and/or clinical practice, along with experts from other disciplines to contribute the chapters.

GENETIC COUNSELING CAN INVOLVE ANYONE AND EVERYONE

Clients attending a genetics clinic may be any age, from newborn babies through to octogenarians. They may be affected with a genetic condition, or at risk of developing one when they are older or passing one on to children. Clients are often distressed, may be facing an uncertain future; they may be terminally ill or bereaved. Clients can be from any ethnic or social group. Some clients may have experience and knowledge of their family's genetic condition; for others, the diagnosis will be brand new. The news of a genetic condition can impact many stages of a client's life, so that the implications of the genetic condition are always with him or her—it is rarely considered "resolved," even for those who test negative for a family condition.

Genetic conditions can be chronic, progressive, life-limiting; the effects of a genetic condition may be obvious at birth, or the onset maybe in young adulthood or middle age. The genetic condition may interfere with the functioning of any system in the body, causing physical and/or learning difficulties. Clients may have dysmorphic features or physical impairments or learning difficulties. Information about genetic conditions is likely to change over time, for example, in terms of our understanding of the phenotype, in the type of molecular testing available, and the health screening and risk management options. Thus, uncertainty reigns for both the client and the genetic healthcare professional.

> In reviewing the medical notes in preparation for a consultation, the genetic health professional may be able to check the latest medical literature to ensure that his or her knowledge of the condition is as up to date as possible, but until he or she meets the client, the professional cannot know how this information may be received and how it will affect the client's life.

Effective counseling requires effective communication: giving information that is relevant to patients' concerns, in a way that is easily understood. (Michie 1994)

"Success" in the genetics clinic is difficult to measure; recent research suggests this relates to the ability to empower clients so that they can make the decisions that are right for them. To achieve this, the genetic health professional should consider all aspects of the communication exchange that he or she facilitates, including recognizing and addressing barriers to communication.

PRACTICAL INFORMATION TO SUPPORT TRANS-/CROSS-CULTURAL COUNSELING

It is absolutely pivotal not to stereotype clients; everyone is different and there is more variation between individuals than among groups of individuals (Wang 2001). However, writers on transcultural counseling do advise that it is helpful to at least have some level of awareness of practical or cultural difference that may exist between counselor and client. Cultural difference can exist on many levels; this does not only relate to ethnicity or race. Healthcare professionals, as individuals, may be very different from the clients they see, and it is helpful to acknowledge rather than ignore this. For example, differences may exist within multiple planes: gender, age, educational background, sexual orientation, religious belief, politics, skin color, physical ability, fluency in language, cultural heritage, and beliefs about genetics. The list is endless. Although it is impossible to know prior to seeing a client what his or her perspective will be, it can at least be helpful if the health professional has given some thought to possible cultural and attitudinal nuances that the client may have.

To become a transculturally skilled counselor, students will need to...attain specific knowledge about the client group/s. (Lago & Thompson 1996)

Numerous genetic counseling books describe the process and techniques of genetic counseling, along with hundreds that describe the specific features of genetic conditions. This book does not aim to delve into any of these issues. Instead, it aims to help genetic health professionals, indeed any health professional, improve their communication with clients by offering practical information and advice about working with specific client groups. Every health professional should already possess a toolkit of good communication skills; our book aims to add another level of awareness that can be incorporated into this toolkit.

We have asked each author, experts in the field, to view his or her chapter as a method for delivery of practical information—we wanted them to imagine they were passing on their worldly advice to another health professional who might, for example, be shadowing them in a consultation. What top tips would they want to impart? What would be considered a "do or a don't"? We were particularly interested in the knowledge that comes from years of experience of working with a particular client group, the subtle cues, the pitfalls, the anticipated outcomes.

We have attempted to identify social and clinical scenarios that may inherently make communication more complex, perhaps due to the exaggerated difference between health professional and client. For example, a health professional who is young may have limited life experience or emotional cues to help him or her relate to a client who is elderly. By the same token, a health professional who is more mature may feel flummoxed by the idea of reaching out and engaging appropriately with a teenager. Due to the fact that genetic counseling may be relevant and appropriate at any stage of life and covers a vast array of different personal and clinical scenarios (as detailed above), it is to be expected that genetic health professionals cannot be expert in all. We have included clinical scenarios in which the genetic health professional might feel unsure of him- or herself or inexperienced in managing a taboo subject, such as talking to a patient who is dying about storing DNA for the future. We have also included cultural scenarios that the genetic health professional may not frequently encounter, for example, working with the Deaf community, Traveller community, or Orthodox Jewish community.

Readers of this book can be at any stage of their genetic counselor or health professional career. The information provided is relevant to students training to be genetic counselors and will also be useful for genetic counselors preparing for registration or certification. In addition, this book aims to be useful for health professionals who are unfamiliar with working within a particular client group and who want to scan the text for some top practical tips. The book has been written in such a way that it can be dipped into and the salient points extracted when a health professional is doing preconsultation preparation. Each chapter is divided into four main sections: Background, Preparing for the Consultation, Communication in the Consultation, and the Summary. The chapter authors have also provided references and suggestions for further reading.

We sincerely hope that readers enjoy this book but, most of all, that they find it useful for their practice.

Jennifer Wiggins and Anna Middleton

REFERENCES

Genetic Counselor Registration Board UK and ROI. (2012). *Code of Conduct*. Available at: www.gcrb.org.uk. (Accessed January 26, 2012.)

Lago, C., & Thompson J. (1996). *Race, culture and counseling*. Buckingham: Open University Press

Michie, S. (1994). Genetic counseling. *Journal of Medical Ethics, 20*, 268–269.

Resta, R., et al. (2006). A new definition of genetic counseling; National Society of Genetic Counselor Task Force Report. *Journal of Genetic Counseling, 15*(2), 77–83.

Wang, O. V. (2001). Multicultural genetic counseling: then now, and in the 21st century. *American Journal of Medical Genetics, 106*, 208–215.

FURTHER READING

Gaff, C. L., and Bylund, C. L. (Eds.). (2010). *Family Communication About Genetics*. Oxford: Oxford University Press.

LeRoy, B., McCarthy Veach, P., & Bartels, D. (Eds.). (2010). *Genetic Counseling Practice: Advanced Concepts and Skills*. Hoboken, NJ: Wiley-Blackwell.

Acknowledgments

The editors would like to acknowledge the support of their employers, the Royal Marsden NHS Foundation Trust, London (Jen Wiggins) and the Wellcome Trust Sanger Institute, Cambridge (Anna Middleton). Anna Middleton would also like to thank the Brocher Foundation in Geneva, Switzerland (www.brocher.ch); it was during a month's residency in 2011 that Anna completed most of her editing work. A special thank you also goes to the Association of Genetic Nurses and Counsellors for supporting the original conference session that inspired this work. Finally, the editors would like to thank their husbands, Barny and Al for keeping the kids busy when quiet time was needed at home to bring this book together.

Contributors

Mushtaq Ahmed, BSc, PGCE, PhD, RGC
Principal Genetic Counselor
Yorkshire Regional Genetics Service
Department of Clinical Genetics
Chapel Allerton Hospital

Alison Clarke RN, RHV, RGC, BSc, MSc
Principal Genetic Counselor
St Mary's Hospital

Nicki Cornwell, BA, MPhil, CQSW
Freelance author

Anna Gregorowski, BSc, MA, RSCN, RGN
Nurse Consultant, Adolescent Health
Great Ormond Street Hospital for Children
NHS Foundation Trust

Georgina Hall, MSc, RGC
Principal Genetic Counselor and Honorary Research Associate
Manchester Academic Health Science Centre
St. Mary's Hospital

Kelly Kohut, MS, CGC, RGC
Genetic Counselor
The Royal Marsden NHS Foundation Trust

Sara Levene, MSc, RGC
Principal Genetic Counselor
Clinical Genetics Department
Guy's and St. Thomas' NHS Foundation Trust

Lih-Mei Liao, PhD, MSc, FBPsS
Consultant Clinical Psychologist & Honorary Reader
UCL Institute for Women's Health
UK

Anna Middleton, PhD, MSc, RGC
Ethics Researcher and Genetic Counselor
Wellcome Trust Sanger Institute
Cambridge

Kathryn Myhill, RN
Genetic Nurse
The Royal Marsden NHS Foundation Trust

Christina Palmer, MS, PhD
Professor
Department of Psychiatry & Biobehavioral Sciences
Department of Human Genetics
University of California, Los Angeles

Alan Phillips, BSc, MSc
Head, Psychosocial Services
Alder Hey Children's NHS Foundation Trust

Margaret Simmonds, BSc, MSc, MA, PhD
UK Androgen Insensitivity Syndrome Support Group

Anna-Marie Stevens, RN, MSc
Macmillan Nurse Consultant Cancer Palliative Care
The Royal Marsden and Royal Brompton Palliative Care Service
The Royal Marsden NHS Foundation Trust

Rachel Taylor, RN, BSc, MSc
Consultant Nurse, Neurogenetics
University College London Hospitals NHS Foundation Trust

Jeremy Turk, MD, BSc, FRCPsych, FRCPCH, DCH
Professor of Developmental Psychiatry
Consultant Child & Adolescent Psychiatrist

Institute of Psychiatry & St. George's University of London
South London & Maudsley Foundation NHS Trust

Jacqueline Turner, MSc, BA, RGC
National Centre for Medical Genetics
Our Lady's Children's Hospital

Jayne Wood, MBBS, MRCP, BSc, PgDip
Consultant Palliative Medicine
The Royal Marsden and Royal Brompton Palliative Care Service
The Royal Marsden NHS Foundation Trust

Jennifer Wiggins, MSc, RGC
Senior Genetic Counsellor
The Royal Marsden NHS Foundation Trust

Getting the Message Across

1 Communicating with Clients Who Are D/deaf or Hard of Hearing

Anna Middleton and Christina Palmer

To effectively communicate, we must realise that we are all different in the way we perceive the world and use this understanding as a guide to our communication with other.
—Anthony Robbins

One child with a genetic deafness is born per thousand children (Morton & Nance 2006), making deafness one of the most common genetic conditions. However, despite this, deaf and hard-of-hearing adults very rarely access genetic counseling services, neither to discuss deafness nor other conditions running through their family (Enns, Boudreault, and Palmer et al. 2010; Middleton et al. 2010a). Many geneticists and genetic counselors assume that deaf adults are not interested in using genetic services. Research has shown that this is not the case (Boudreault et al. 2010), but deaf people face many barriers; these include problems with communication, misunderstandings about what genetic counseling is, and difficulties in arranging a referral due to anxieties about how to explain this to referring doctors, as well as worries about a lack of Deaf Awareness (see later) on the part of the health professionals (Middleton et al. 2010b).

Many healthcare professionals do not know the specific communication techniques they need to employ to converse effectively with deaf people, and this has led to a very poor experience on the part of many deaf clients; thus, interactions with the healthcare service in general are known to be severely unsatisfactory (Dye & Kyle 2001; Reeves & Kokoruwe 2005; RNID 2004; Steinberg et al. 2006). General frustrations that deaf people have with regards to the health service appear to influence their preconceived ideas about genetic services (Middleton 2009a). It is widely known that some deaf people have a distrust of health professionals, coupled with a real anxiety about using health services. In addition to this distrust, there are often concerns about the perceived misuses of genetic testing (Middleton et al. 1998; Martinez, Linden, Schimmenti, & Palmer 2003) and an apprehension about interacting with genetic professionals. However, when given accurate information about what genetic counseling is and how to seek out a referral, deaf adults are keen to connect with genetic services (Middleton et al. 2010a).

This chapter aims to offer practical information to help genetic professionals engage effectively with deaf clients. It covers background information about deafness and its impact on individuals and families. It shows how to prepare for a consultation, what sort of interpreter should be arranged, how to book an interpreter, and what sorts of issues are important to deaf people within a genetic consultation. Finally, it covers Deaf Awareness and how communication should be facilitated so that accessibility and communication are optimal for the deaf client.

BACKGROUND

Clients Who are Deaf or Hard of Hearing

Deafness can be highly variable and can affect individuals in different ways. Someone with an audiogram classification in the profound or a severe range would normally find it challenging to hear conversational speech. The terms *profound, severe, moderate,* and *mild* "deafness" have precise audiological definitions that describe the level of hearing loss with respect to sounds used in conversational speech (Prosser & Martini 2007). Hearing impairment may change over time or may be static. Individuals can be deaf due to a variety of reasons; the most common gene that plays a part in nonsyndromic deafness is *GJB2*, also known as Connexin 26 (this latter term refers to the protein made by the GJB2 gene). This (typically) recessive gene has a carrier frequency of approximately 1 in 33, and homozygotes for *GJB2* (as well as biallelic carriers for *GJB2/GJB6*) usually have a severe-profound, congenital hearing loss, although some individuals have audiograms that fall in the mild or moderate range (Smith & Van Camp 2010). Because the focus on this book is on communication within a clinic, no further attention will be given here to the genetic causes of deafness or to a clinical overview; the interested reader is directed to comprehensive texts provided by experts in the field, such as Smith and Van Camp at the GeneReviews section of the www.genetests.org website.

Terms That Deaf People Use to Describe Themselves

There is often disparity in the terminology linked with deafness, largely because people with hearing loss and health professionals and academics use different terms to describe similar concepts (Grundfast & Rosen 1992).

"Hearing impaired" has a precise medical description, as defined by the International Classification of Functioning, Disability, and Health (Stephens & Danermark 2005) and, as such, is often used by health professionals. However, many deaf people themselves do not like this term because it has a negative connotation (as if the person him- or herself were defective or "impaired"). It is therefore not seen as politically correct, and several professional organizations (such as the Royal National Institute for Deaf People [RNID] in the United Kingdom) and representatives for deaf people have dropped the use of this term. Therefore, within a genetic consultation, direct communication with a deaf client should not involve use of the term "hearing impaired" unless the client him- or herself uses it.

There has been a push recently to avoid using a medical condition to describe a person (e.g., "the breast cancer client"). It is seen as more politically correct to refer to the person first and the condition second (e.g., "the client with breast cancer"). This phraseology does not completely translate to deafness because the term "deaf" can often be linked to identity (as will be shown later, in sections on medical versus cultural identity). For example, it is still perfectly acceptable and indeed preferable to use the descriptor "deaf people" rather than "people with deafness." However, for those who don't perceive themselves as deaf but more as having started out hearing and lost some or all of this function, then the phrases "person with hearing loss," "person who is partially hearing," "person with hearing impairment" are acceptable (see Figure 1.1).

Often, the term "deaf" (written with a lowercase d) is used generically to refer to all those with a hearing loss, including those who were born deaf as well as those who began life hearing and have lost this over time. In this chapter, the term "deafness" and "deaf people" is used collectively to refer to people with any level and perception of hearing loss.

Medical or Cultural Model?

Medical Model

- The medical model perceives deafness as a medical problem or pathology due to a deficit within the ear that needs to be treated with a hearing aid or cochlear implant. Health professionals (e.g., audiologists and ear, nose, and throat [ENT] surgeons) traditionally work within the medical model and may assume that the deaf client wishes to be treated or cured of his or her deafness. However, genetic professionals need to be aware that deaf clients coming for genetic counseling may not perceive their deafness from the medical model.
- People who perceive their hearing loss from the medical perspective usually use spoken language and identify more with the Hearing World (also termed "culturally hearing"). They also may believe that they have a disability and, within

People who are 'Hard of Hearing':
- May have mild-moderate hearing loss
- Often derive use from hearing aid
- Often spoken language user
- Often culturally hearing

In this chapter 'hard of hearing' is used to refer to people who started out hearing and who have become deaf or lost their hearing over time

People who are 'Deafened':
- May have profound deafness
- Loss may be sudden and/or progressive
- May derive little use from hearing aid
- Usually spoken language user
- Mostly culturally hearing

People who are 'deaf':
- May have severe-profound deafness
- May be spoken language user but might include sign language user
- 'deaf' may denote culturally hearing, but if used generically may include culturally Deaf
In this text 'deaf' is used in two contexts, firstly to refer to people who are NOT culturally Deaf.
Secondly as generic term for everyone
- 'deaf' can include those who are hard of hearing, Deaf and deafened.

'deaf community' is a generic term to include everyone (e.g. hard of hearing people, deafened and Deaf people)

People who are 'Deaf':
- Usually have profound deafness
- May/May not derive use from hearing aids
- Are sign language users
- Are culturally Deaf

In this chapter, 'Deaf' is used exclusively to refer to people who use sign language as their first language and who consider themselves Culturally Deaf.
'Deaf' community is a specific term that refers to people who are culturally Deaf sign language users

FIGURE 1.1
Terminology and Broad Descriptors.

a genetic counseling context, may be keen to avoid passing on deafness to their children.

Cultural Model

- The cultural or linguistic model determines that deafness is a way of life rather than a medical problem that requires treatment.
- People who are culturally deaf use signed language as their preferred communication and often refer to themselves as Deaf (written with an uppercase D) (Padden & Humphries 2005); these clients define themselves as part of the Deaf community or Deaf World. They may believe that they do not have a disability, but that society disables them. Within a genetic counseling context, they may not mind passing on deafness to their children.

- When several members of the same family have deafness and use sign language as their preferred language, a strong Deaf identity often develops. It is thought that 90% of culturally Deaf adults have a Deaf rather than a hearing partner (Schein 1989); 70% of D/deaf couples who have only deaf children are believed to be deaf because of changes to the GJB2 gene (Nance et al. 2000).
- The "Deaf culture" is worldwide, and there are many active Deaf communities, for example, in the United States, United Kingdom, Australia, Canada, Germany, Sweden, the Netherlands, and elsewhere.

Different Perceptions of Deafness

- A person who is hard of hearing or deafened will usually perceive his or her deafness from the medical model and will usually use spoken language, lipreading, and written forms to communicate. He or she may feel incredibly disabled by the hearing loss and may have to make significant practical and emotional adjustments in his or her life to adapt to this.
- A person who considers him- or herself culturally Deaf may reject the medical model of deafness; he or she usually uses a National Sign Language (e.g., British Sign Language [BSL] or American Sign Language [ASL]) to communicate, with some lipreading; because spoken English is a second language, some may prefer not to use written/read English. These individuals often feel pride attached to their deafness and, in many circumstances, express a preference to being deaf rather than hearing (Ladd 2003).

Different Ways Deaf People Communicate

Deaf and hard-of-hearing people can use several different methods of communication. These include (but are not limited to) speech; National Signed Language (e.g., BSL, ASL); Signed Supported Spoken Language (SSSL), which translates spoken language into sign language using the same word order and structure as the spoken language (e.g., Signed Supported English); lip- or speech-reading; and written notes.

Spoken Language

The vast majority of hard-of-hearing and deafened people use spoken language. Within this, they may rely heavily on lipreading and a strong level of Deaf Awareness on the part of the person with whom they are communicating (Middleton et al. 2010b). Conversely, lipreading for a profoundly deaf person who has never heard sound can be incredibly challenging (Barnett 2002). It is possible for different words to look the same to a person who is lip-reading; this is because in spoken language it is the sound made within the throat (which is thus invisible to the viewer) that identifies the differences between words. For example, "fifteen" and "fifty" look almost identical to a lipreader (Harmer 1999).

> When communicating with people who are lip-reading, it is vital not to obscure the face, as with fingers or a pen. It is also very important to maintain eye contact because the person lip-reading will be looking not only at the mouth, but also at the jaw, cheeks, and eyes and getting cues from facial expressions and animation. It is also hugely helpful if the person being lip-read offers signposting within the conversation, for example, "I'm going to ask you about your deafness first and then you can tell me about your relatives."

Many deaf people who have had significant speech therapy input may give the impression of good spoken language by using clear speech with good voice control. However, this might be misleading in that they may not be able to follow and understand speech with the same ease (see Box 1.1).

> It should never be assumed that a deaf person comprehends everything spoken to him or her, and it is important to check frequently for understanding and to use different methods for getting the same message across. This can be done using repetition and rehearsal (i.e., repeating the same concept but using different words: "I'm going to take your family tree," "I'm going to ask you about your family history," "I'd like to learn more about your family and who is deaf." If it is obvious that a particular sentence is causing confusion, it is important not to just repeat it more loudly, but to rephrase it in several different ways.

Box 1.1 Case Study 1: Working with a Lip-Speaker

Mr. and Mrs. Brown are both severely deaf; so too are their two teenage daughters. The family uses speech to communicate; all wear hearing aids and refer to themselves as "hard of hearing" rather than by any other terms. They were referred for genetic counseling because Mr. Brown participated in a research project through one of the deafness support groups and discovered that he was a homozygote for the 35delG mutation in the GJB2 gene. His wife was very keen to have genetic testing for herself and their daughters. Prior to the clinic, the genetic counselor contacted the family via telephone. She used the British Telecom relay service, TypeTalk, which enables communication with deaf people through a hearing operator who converts speech into text, which is then received via the deaf person's computer. Once she started to communicate with Mr. and Mrs. Brown, they informed her that they preferred to use MSN Messenger, and so the genetic counselor arranged to have a direct text-based conversation instead.

Mr. and Mrs. Brown said that they would like a "communication supporter" called a "lip-speaker" at their consultation. They had worked previously with a lip-speaker they liked, and they provided the name and contact details so that the genetic counselor could contact her. The genetic counselor booked this lip-speaker and sent her details of the sorts of issues that would be discussed in the consultation, together with an explanation of some genetic terminology she would be using. The genetic counselor arranged to meet the lip-speaker 20 minutes prior to the consultation, so that they could arrange the chairs appropriately in the room in relation to the light and also have a chat about how the genetic counselor would conduct the session. The genetic counselor asked the lip-speaker to speak to the receptionist for the clinic and to make arrangements to be brought over to the reception as soon as Mr. and Mrs. Brown made themselves known. This meant that the lip-speaker would be able to sit with Mr. and Mrs. Brown and their children in the waiting area and alert them when the genetic counselor was ready to see them. When the genetic counselor called out their names, the Brown family was prompted by the lip-speaker that it was their turn, and the family came into the consultation room. The session started with the family checking that the seating arrangements were suitable for them; the lip-speaker sat to the genetic counselor's side, so that all the family could lip-read the genetic counselor and look to the lip-speaker easily for prompts. The genetic counselor conducted the session, and the lip-speaker mouthed the English clearly together with finger-spelled letters for individual words. The genetic counselor took her time, took care not to use jargon, and repeated and rephrased what she said, because this is particularly useful for lipreading. She also paused between changes in topic and checked periodically that the lip-speaker was keeping up. Effective communication was delivered in speech via the support of the lip-speaker, and the deaf family was able to engage fully in their genetic counseling consultation because of this.

Note: In the United States, deaf individuals who prefer to use speech might use TTY service or MSN Messenger service for direct communication with their genetic counselor.

National Sign Language

National Sign Languages (NSL) have their own systems of grammar and sentence construction that is different from—and not a literal translation of—spoken languages (Fischer & Hulst 2003). National Sign Languages vary among countries; for example, the sign language in the United States is different from BSL; there are also regional dialects within countries. A person using an NSL would not usually use his or her voice to speak at the same time, but he or she may mouth some individual words. This is different from SSSL, in which the signing is based literally on the spoken language. People who are culturally Deaf would usually use an NSL rather than a SSSL.

Sign Supported Spoken Language

For deaf children born into hearing families, an emphasis may be placed on developing spoken language. These deaf children also may learn to sign via SSSL because SSSL has the same sentence construction as spoken language. SSSL may also be used by deaf and hard-of-hearing people who would not consider themselves culturally Deaf but who span the Deaf and Hearing Worlds. Sign language interpreters often are trained to recognize whether a deaf individual is using SSSL (a coded form of spoken language) or an NSL (a signed language) and will adapt their signing and voicing accordingly.

Reading/Writing

Deaf people who use NSLs may find reading and writing more difficult than do SSSL users because the written form of a language has the same sentence construction as SSSL, rather than NSL. Thus, it may not be helpful to use written notes with an NSL user (although in some cases, for the sake of confidentiality, an NSL user may prefer using written notes rather than a sign language interpreter as a means of communication with a healthcare provider—it is important to ascertain a Deaf individual's preferred mode of communication prior to an appointment). It also means that written text by an NSL user may give the impression that English is a second language (which, of course, it is!); for example, sentences may contain differently ordered grammar or spelling mistakes. It is very important to realize that this is in no way indicative of intellectual ability but is rather a symbol of difficulties in receiving the most suitable education to facilitate multilingual achievement. Where written material is the only available medium, it is important to have this structured in "Plain English" for sign language users, and there are companies that specialize in this work. Plain English is a written form of English in which care has been taken to reduce sentence size, restrict the use of jargon, and avoid legal-speak. The British government places particular emphasis on the fact that all publications produced for the lay person be written in lay language that is easy to understand.

> Where possible, written materials (e.g., clinic information) should be translated into sign language with captioned text and offered in an electronic form (e.g., on DVD). Consideration also needs to be given to the way consent forms and family history questionnaires are formulated and could also be delivered in a signed electronic format.

Genetic Counseling Isn't Always About Deafness

A client with hearing loss may come for genetic counseling for the same reasons that hearing clients do, so genetic professionals need to remove the common mindset that deaf clients are only interested in genetic counseling for deafness. Although discussing deafness may be something that some Deaf and hard-of-hearing people are very interested in, there are also many who are quite simply tired of this being the only conversation they seem to have when they meet health professionals. If a Deaf client comes for genetic counseling because of a family history of breast cancer or to discuss prenatal testing for cystic fibrosis, then the genetic counselor needs to be mindful to focus the consultation on that topic.

> It is common for Deaf people to feel that they are a "curiosity" to (well-intentioned) others who simply want to quiz them about their language and ability to adapt to a hearing world.

Having Children

Those Deaf and hard-of-hearing people who are interested in knowing more about the inheritance of deafness in their family may wish to know about passing on deafness to children because they may prefer to have deaf rather than hearing children (Middleton et al. 2001). For some families, deafness is something that they wish to avoid at all costs; to others, having deaf children is preferred (Dolnick 1993; Erting 1994; Hoffmeister 1985; Middleton et al. 1998). Conversely, when a deaf baby is born into a hearing family, the experience can be devastating, and hearing parents may grieve extensively for the fact that their child cannot hear (Meadow 1980).

Historical Context to Deafness, Eugenics, and Genetics

Assuming that all deaf couples will have deaf children (an inaccurate assumption) has led eugenicists throughout history to create policy that prevented deaf couples from having children (Schuchman 2004). Within relatively recent history, the deaf community was a specific group targeted for enforced sterilization and euthanasia under the Nazi regime (Schuchman 2004). This persecution at the hands of hearing people is something the Deaf community holds in their history and culture.

> The words *genetics* and *eugenics* sound and look similar (in signed language), and even today, when deaf people are asked to give their views on genetics, they often mention eugenic principles and assume that modern-day genetic services encourage the routine abortion of deaf fetuses (Middleton et al. 2010a). Genetic professionals *must* be aware of the history of persecution that deaf people have faced in the name of eugenics, and that deaf and hard-of-hearing people still associate this past with modern genetic services.

When deaf and hard-of-hearing people were asked what they thought genetic counseling is, there tended to be two camps—those who thought it must involve some kind of therapeutic counseling for mental health issues, and those who thought it must involve prenatal testing for deafness with recommended selective abortion (Middleton et al. 2010a).

The power of this latter issue should not be underestimated because it may hinder engagement with genetic services. For example, a deaf client may decline a prenatal test for Duchenne muscular dystrophy because he or she wrongly assumes that deafness will also be tested for at the same time.

It is, therefore, incredibly helpful to start any genetic counseling consultation with a brief description of what the consultation will entail and what the genetic counseling process involves (see Box 1.2).

Box 1.2 Case Study 2: Working with Assumptions About Genetic Counseling

Mrs. Smith is profoundly deaf. She is also culturally Deaf and British Sign Language (BSL) is her first language. She does not wear a hearing aid nor have a cochlear implant, and her lipreading skills are adequate, but she finds it difficult to fully comprehend a full conversation via lipreading. Mrs. Smith is pregnant and, on the routine 20-week scan, it was found that the fetus had echogenic bowel, together with other features that could be indicative of cystic fibrosis. The prenatal genetic counselor became involved with Mrs. Smith because she was referred to discuss cystic fibrosis and the pros and cons of having a diagnostic chorionic villus sampling (CVS) (the center she went to routinely performed CVS throughout pregnancy, not just in the first trimester). The genetic counselor was informed by the referring obstetrician that Mrs. Smith is Deaf and preferred to be contacted via text on her mobile telephone. The genetic counselor sent a text to Mrs. Smith to ask what sort of interpreter she preferred and whether she had any preferences for who was booked. Mrs. Smith said that she needed a BSL interpreter and that anyone from the Signature website (U.K. based) would be appropriate. Mrs. Smith also said that, because she could access e-mail on her phone, she would prefer to continue the conversation via e-mail so that more could be discussed. Over the next two days, arrangements were made via e-mail for the consultation and the interpreter. The genetic counselor was careful to compose short messages about what would be discussed in the clinic (e.g., a discussion about the ultrasound findings and the possibility of additional testing), because this text-based communication was in written English—not Mrs. Smith's first language—and thus there was room for possible misunderstanding. The genetic counselor was also aware that Mrs. Smith may be very nervous about undergoing prenatal testing and may wrongly assume that deafness would be tested for. This hunch was correct, and, within the consultation, Mrs. Smith revealed that she had reservations about going ahead with prenatal genetic diagnosis for cystic fibrosis and wanted additional reassurance that deafness would not be tested for. She was particularly suspicious that the obstetricians would encourage a termination of pregnancy if the baby was thought to be deaf. The genetic counselor was able to reassure Mrs. Smith that this would not happen; by facilitating Mrs. Smiths' preferred communication channels (text, e-mail, interpreter), the genetic counselor was able to address many of Mrs. Smith's fears and preconceived ideas about the process of genetic counseling.

Note: Although this example focuses on a British Deaf client, the essential point about the importance of facilitating the preferred communication channels holds worldwide. In many countries (e.g., Britain, United States), it is a legal requirement that sign language interpreters be available when requested by a deaf client. Moreover, a genetic service can build rapport and illustrate Deaf Awareness by asking a sign language user if he or she has a preference for a specific sign language interpreter or agency when booking a sign language interpreter. If a genetic service or medical center has a sign language interpreter on staff, this should be explained in advance to the Deaf client so that he or she understands why the genetic counselor or genetic staff did not ask for suggestions.

PREPARING FOR THE CONSULTATION

Disability legislation in a variety of countries (for example, the Disability Discrimination Act in the United Kingdom; the Americans with Disabilities Act in the United States) decrees that it is the service provider's responsibility to ensure that appropriate measures are taken to enable equal access to services for deaf and hard-of-hearing clients; the service provider also must cover the cost of this.

One way to ensure equal access is to employ the services of a Deaf Awareness or Deaf Equality consultancy service (usually run by Deaf advocates who are able to advise on the most appropriate way to deliver services) to assess what is available and make recommendations. Cultural awareness is another important aspect of genetic services for Deaf clients. Genetic services providers, including genetic counselors, can develop cultural awareness through a series of Deaf culture workshops and by developing ties with local and national Deaf organizations.

The Clinic Booking Process

Any clinic booking process that relies on the client phoning the hospital or service to book or confirm an appointment is difficult for a deaf or hard-of-hearing client.

Communication with deaf clients needs to be adapted; this can be done using e-mail, texting, or through online messenger services (e.g., MSN Messenger) (Baldwin et al. 2011; Withrow et al. 2009).

The Waiting Room

Waiting for your name to be called out prior to a consultation is one of the most stressful events for a deaf client: thousands of health service appointments have been missed because the deaf person didn't hear his or her name being called. When the deaf client arrives for his or her appointment, the reception staff need to know that they must adapt their communication style. Staff should be encouraged to take a Deaf Awareness training course: they need to speak clearly, use good Deaf Awareness skills (see later), and inform the client how he or she will know when it is his or her turn for the appointment. Several different methods can work. A visual board that displays the client's name (either written or electronic) and where to go can be useful. However, as with calling out a client's name, this does breach confidentiality. Alternatively, each client could be given a number on a piece of paper, and the genetic counsellor can then hold up the number corresponding to the client when it is his or her turn. Since clinic clients generally must sign in when they arrive at the clinic, another option is for the staff to be aware of the day(s) on which a deaf client has an appointment. Staff can meet the deaf client as he or she signs in, walk over to the deaf client when it is his or her appointment time, and walk him or her to the assigned clinic room. Another option is to use a vibrating pager, which the client holds while waiting; it vibrates when it is his or her turn. This latter method is particularly appropriate for deaf clients because it doesn't rely on them keeping a very firm look out for visual cues; it means they can relax while they are waiting. For hearing aid users, the inclusion of an induction loop is pivotal.

It is also very important to appreciate that deaf clients cannot easily communicate if they cannot easily see—sending them off to a busy waiting room with plants, tables, and people standing around can be incredibly stressful if they cannot easily view the visual notice board or genetic professional who has come to get them. Simple things like moving chairs so that they face the space where the genetic professional will stand can make all the difference.

Observations of the Deaf Client Before the Consultation Starts

Seeing a hearing aid on a deaf client may offer some clues as to how he or she prefers to communicate. It is possible that he or she utilizes his or her residual hearing and thus will use lipreading and spoken language. Alternatively, he or she may be a sign language user predominantly but gain some helpful cues from the hearing aid (but not enough to actually "hear" a conversation in its entirety). It should not be assumed that, if no hearing aid is seen, the client is not deaf; such clients may be sign language users and gain no useful benefit from a hearing aid.

Timing of Consultations

The time taken for a routine genetic counseling consultation could be doubled for a deaf client. When an interpreter is used, time needs to be allowed for the interpreter to listen to what is being said and translate this into sign language, for the deaf client to watch this and then respond in sign language, and for the sign language interpreter to translate the response into spoken language. The messages being delivered by the genetic counselor need to be repeatedly rephrased and delivered in different ways, to allow the deaf client the chance to overcome inevitable obstacles with lip-reading or to allow the sign language interpreter the chance to overcome inevitable obstacles with translating genetic and medical terminology (unfamiliar to most interpreters) into sign language.

> It is usual and natural for consultations to take more time with deaf and hard-of-hearing clients. It is also necessary to allow for a short break during a consultation. This is because it is particularly tiring following a translated conversation, as well as trying to lip-read and also sometimes deal with distracting ambient noise at the same time. Genetic counselors should also be aware that many deaf and hard-of-hearing people have tinnitus (ringing in the ears) that can be incredibly distracting and also can make stressful situations even worse with regards to being able to concentrate.

Preferences for Communication in a Clinical Setting

Research has shown that many deaf sign language users prefer their healthcare consultations to be delivered in sign language, preferably by a signing health professional or, if that is not possible, then via an interpreter (Baldwin et al. 2011; Dye & Kyle 2001; Middleton et al. 2010b; Withrow et al. 2009). However, if a signing health professional is not available, some deaf sign language users will prefer their healthcare consultations to be conducted using written communication rather than via an interpreter. This is because they do not wish to have a third party (sign language interpreter) privy to their medical information; they prefer to keep their medical information between themselves and their healthcare provider. Sign language users are usually resistant to consultations delivered only in speech, and it is the clinicians' responsibility to ensure that the appropriate methods of communication (e.g., interpreters) are in place.

Hard-of-hearing spoken language users are accepting of consultations in speech but only if there is a good level of Deaf Awareness on the part of the genetic professional (Middleton et al. 2010b); this may mean also using handwritten notes and electronic note-taking, and time needs to be allowed for the client to switch his or her gaze from reading the written notes and to the genetic professional for lipreading.

Types of Interpreter and Communication Support

Information can be interpreted in several different ways, depending on the preferences of the deaf or hard-of-hearing client. An *interpreter* will turn an NSL or SSSL into spoken language, and spoken language into an NSL or SSSL. A *communication support professional* (e.g., a *lip-speaker*) will turn spoken language into clear spoken language accessible to both the hearing health professional and the deaf or hard-of-hearing client. A *speech-to-text reporter* (STTR) and *voice-to-text software* convert speech into written text (available on many computers and smart phones). *Deaf relay interpreters* work with hearing interpreters; they convert the sign language used by the hearing interpreters into a tailor-made sign language for the deaf client. As an example, a deaf interpreter fluent in BSL would be used for a deaf client whose native language is BSL but is receiving genetic services in the United States via a hearing interpreter trained in ASL. All these services can be available in person or via an online service.

For some individuals, expressive and receptive language will be the same. Others may prefer to express themselves through spoken language but receive information in a signed language.

Before the consultation begins, it is most helpful to ask the deaf or hard-of-hearing client what form of communication support they prefer. They may also have a particular person whom they prefer to work with, or, alternatively, a particular gender of interpreter (e.g., if the consultation will involve a physical examination). Interpreters are often well known in the Deaf community and may also be hearing children of deaf parents themselves; thus, it is distinctly possible that the deaf client may know the interpreter socially and may feel quite strongly about working with (or not with) certain interpreters.

It is not thought good practice to allow a younger child or relative to be used as an interpreter. It is always the responsibility of the genetic service to pay the cost of the interpreter, as well as travel expenses and booking fee (if there is one). For a more comprehensive overview of the different types of interpreters available see www. signature.org.uk (in the United Kingdom), www.rid.org (in the United States), and www.deafau.org.au (in Australia).

Working with Interpreters

Once the most appropriate interpreter or communication support person has been booked, it is important to put aside some time, ahead of the consultation, to speak with them about the content of the consultation. Ideally, this would happen several days before meeting in person, but when this isn't possible, it should definitely be scheduled for at least half an hour before the consultation. This is because the interpreter needs to have time to practice how he or she will relay certain concepts, and it is also likely that he or she will want to double-check meanings and intentions with the genetic professional to make the communication as clear as possible. With a complicated subject like genetic, it is imperative that the genetic counselor spends time explaining the biology behind, for example, inheritance patterns, so that the interpreter can prepare what sort of visual metaphors he or she may use and check these out. It is often helpful to send diagrams or explanations ahead of the consultation. If bad news is going to be given, then it is helpful to give the interpreter some warning of this—not necessarily to give the news before the client receives it, but to forewarn the interpreter of the sorts of issues that may arise so that he or she is not caught off guard. An important balance must be struck between preparing an interpreter for a session and ensuring that the interpreter does not receive distinctly personal information about the deaf client before the deaf client receives that same information. This balance should be rigorously respected; otherwise (1) it is possible that the information will affect the interpreter's demeanor and disrupt the healthcare professional's plan for conducting the session, and (2) if the deaf client decides to cancel the appointment, then the interpreter is left knowing something very significant about the deaf client without that deaf client's knowledge, which could create ethical dilemmas.

Sometimes, the client may prefer for the interpreter to meet him or her in the waiting area and come into the clinic with the client. Thus, it is imperative that decisions are made about what preparation the interpreter needs and what the client expects so that all are clear on what will be happening. When the interpreter and client are present in the consultation room, there will likely be a discussion about the seating and how this is positioned in relation to the light; chairs may be moved around and it is up to the genetic counselor to make sure that everyone is seated in a position where he or she can easily be seen by both interpreter and client.

It is important for the genetic counselor not to assume that every message he or she wishes to relay through the interpreter is actually relayed word for word and with the same intonation and tone intended. There is nearly always some difficulty encountered at some point. It is therefore important not to speak too fast and to keep an eye on the interpreter to check that he or she appears to be keeping up. It is also important to pause frequently to allow time for the interpreter to catch up and also to pause between changes in topic so that the interpreter can indicate to the deaf client that a new set of information is on its way.

> It is important for the genetic counselor to "control" the session. If the client needs comforting, it is for the genetic counselor to do this, not the interpreter.

Sign language interpreters will also interpret other people's conversations or sounds (e.g., telephone, music) if they hear it. Since hearing people have access to these "extraneous" sounds, it is perfectly acceptable for deaf people to also have access. Thus, if a genetic counselor's phone rings in the middle of the session, and she chooses to answer it and have a conversation, the interpreter will alert the deaf client that the phone is ringing and will interpret what the genetic counselor is saying over the phone (which is no different from a hearing client having access to the genetic counselor's phone conversation), even though this conversation has nothing to do with the current session.

The process of interpreting means that the interpreter makes sense of what the client is expressing; this may mean that sometimes the interpreter "fills in the gaps" as he or she translates what he or she thinks the deaf client is expressing. Although this always involves a level of intuition and empathy, there are also occasions when what the Deaf client is expressing is not well understood by the interpreter. It is also distinctly possible that what the Deaf client is expressing is incoherent or muddled (e.g., if he or she has a mental health issue); thus, the interpreter will often have to make an immediate judgment on whether to express his or her own interpretation of what is being communicated, whether he or she interprets "a flavor" of this, or whether a literal translation (that may make no sense) is most appropriate. For these reasons, it is therefore vitally important to have a debriefing session with the interpreter after a consultation, to check that the interpreter was satisfied with the exchange of language and that there was nothing missing.

Booking an Interpreter

There is no universally recognized register of interpreters; however, most countries will have their own accredited organizations for interpreting, and so it is helpful to do an Internet search to learn about the accreditation requirements in a specific country. Many hospitals will have access to particular interpreting agencies; however, since a different interpreter is usually sent for each assignment, many health professionals prefer to establish their own network of interpreters that they like to work with. Limiting the pool allows chosen interpreters an opportunity to build expertise.

> A consultation that is likely to last more than an hour may require two interpreters; they usually work for 20–30 minutes and then swap over.

It is important to allow several weeks to book an interpreter to attend a consultation in person. However, it is possible to gain access to instant, live online BSL interpreting via the Internet, for example at www.signtranslate.com. If an online interpreter is required, the same rules apply in that it is important to allow time to prepare the interpreter for the language and concepts that will be discussed in the consultation. When booking an interpreter, the following information will be required: nature of consultation (medical), number of deaf people and number of hearing people in the consultation, where the consultation is (directions to be sent), the content of the consultation (preparation material to be sent, such as explanations of what recessive inheritance is and an overview of the topics for discussion), who the deaf client(s) is, how long the consultation will last, where exactly to meet (e.g., in the waiting room with the deaf client or the clinic room before the deaf client arrives, etc.).

The following is from the British Deaf Association guide on working with interpreters (British Deaf Association 2005, www.bda.org.uk):

- "Talk directly to the Deaf person. Correct: 'Did you have trouble finding us today?' Incorrect: 'Please ask if s/he had trouble finding us today?'
- The spoken side of the interpretation is called the 'voice-over' and will always be in first person, e.g.: 'I had no trouble finding you; your directions were very clear.' The Deaf person is 'speaking' with the interpreter's voice.
- Look at the Deaf person and not the interpreter. Maintaining good eye contact will reinforce the feeling of direct communication.
- The interpreter will not take part in the discussion, and is impartial. During the communication, do not ask an interpreter for their opinion or advice.
- The interpreter relays what they hear, so the Deaf person has full access to all communication. Do not say anything you don't want everyone to know!
- The interpreter will interrupt if they need something to be repeated or clarified. Equally, if you are not sure of something, you can ask the Deaf person to repeat or rephrase it. If you think the interpreter may have misunderstood or missed something, it's fine to ask to go back and find out for sure.
- Position the interpreter close to the main speaker if possible, and clearly visible to the Deaf person. The interpreter should be well lit, but not from behind—so do not put them in front of a bright window!
- Don't be put off if the Deaf person doesn't watch you when you are talking, because they'll be watching the interpreter.
- The interpreter can only listen to or watch one person at a time, so—as with any communication—it is important to take turns and not talk over each other.
- Speak clearly at your normal pace. Interpretation is almost simultaneous, but there will be a slight delay as the interpreter picks up the meaning of a phrase. If you usually speak very quickly, you may need to slow down a little (the interpreter can advise you). Allow time for Deaf people to respond or ask questions.

• Afterwards, as part of the feedback process, check with the Deaf person whether interpreting arrangements were satisfactory, and whether they would be happy to use the same interpreter again. If you have suggestions for improvement, tell the interpreter or the agency."

Deaf Awareness

"Deaf Awareness" is the conscious attention given to making sure that communication is appropriate and sensitive to the deaf client's needs. This means adapting one's communication style to the individual client—all deaf and hard-of-hearing people are different and may have slightly different needs. For example, an elderly hearing aid user might find it helpful if his or her genetic professional slowed down his or her speech and also raised it slightly. Conversely, this is unlikely to be at all helpful for someone who is good at lipreading and who has a finely tuned hearing aid—the slowed speech distorts lipreading and the hearing aid warps the sound if it is too loud. The following text gives details of good Deaf Awareness for sign language and spoken language users (see Figures 1.2 and 1.3).

Training Recommendations for Staff Working in Genetic Services

• Substantial Deaf Awareness training is recommended for at least one member of administration staff and one member of clinical staff in each genetics department. This training should be offered by someone who is deaf, or if this is not feasible, training should have significant input from someone who is deaf.

Greeting
>   Welcome the client with a sign-language greeting (or ask the client to teach you one)
>   Ask the client how best to communicate with him or her

Environment
>   Room is well lit, and the light is not shining in the client's eyes
>   People are positioned so that the client who is deaf can see the doctor and the interpreter

Expressive communication
>   Work with a qualified interpreter
>   Speak to the client, not the interpreter
>   Topic changes are stated explicitly
>   Note writing and written materials may have limited usefulness
>   Ask the client periodically about the quality of the communication
>   Ask the client for periodic summaries to check accuracy of communication

Receptive communication
>   Look at the client while listening to the interpreter
>   When uncertain, ask the client (not the interpreter) for clarification
>   Summarise the client's story to check accuracy
>   (Barnett 2002, p696)

FIGURE 1.2
Deaf Awareness for Deaf Sign Language Users.

Greeting

> Ask the client how best to communicate with him or her

Environment

> Background noise is minimized
> [Health professional's] face is well lit

Expressive communication

> Eye contact is established before speaking
> View of mouth is not obscured (by hands, pens, charts etc)
> Adjust voice pitch if this helps
> Topic changes are stated explicitly
> Repeat information that is not understood. Rephrase if it is still not understood
> Use assistive listening devices (e.g. hearing aids, note-takers) if they help
> Note writing may be helpful
> Ask the client periodically about the quality of the communication
> Ask the client for periodic summaries to check accuracy of communication

Receptive communication

> When uncertain, ask the client to repeat or clarify
> Repeat the client's statement to confirm comprehension
> If still unclear, note writing may help
> Summarise the client's story to check accuracy
> (Barnett 2002, p695-6)

FIGURE 1.3

Deaf Awareness for Hard-of-Hearing Spoken Language Users.

- All genetic professionals who regularly see deaf and hard-of-hearing clients (e.g., on a monthly basis) should have Deaf Awareness training.
- At least one member of the genetic team frequently seeing deaf sign language users (e.g., as part of a specialist deafness clinic, perhaps on a monthly or even weekly basis) should undertake NSL training at least to a basic level.
- Genetic professionals who specialize in working with deaf clients and who frequently see deaf sign language users should aim for fluency in their NSL and be able to deliver a consultation in NSL (Middleton 2009b).

Marking of Medical Records

Medical notes should be clearly labeled with the communication needs of a deaf or hard-of-hearing client. This may mean printing in bold on the front page or the notes or adding an auto-alert to electronic records that indicates the client is, for example, "profoundly deaf," "uses British Sign Language," and "prefers to use Mr. X, BSL interpreter from Y agency (telephone number…)."

Use of Language

Value-laden terms should not be used to give deafness a negative connotation (e.g., avoid "mutation," "abnormal," "normal," be sensitive to words like "risk"). Words such as "chromosome," "gene," and "DNA" may need to be finger-spelled and have a definition applied. This is why it is helpful for the interpreter to have been given the opportunity to learn for him- or herself what these terms mean before the consultation; they can then think creatively about how they will describe this in sign language.

Taking a Family History

Deaf children growing up in hearing families often miss out on incidental conversations that occur within the family because of communication difficulties. This means that they may have a lack of knowledge about relatives and their medical conditions. Therefore, when taking a family history, it may be necessary to get permission to call hearing relatives to gather more information (Israel & Arnos 1995). Other options from our experience are (1) ask the deaf client to ask his or her hearing relatives to assist in filling out a family history questionnaire, and (2) ask the deaf client to text his or her hearing relatives with family history questions as they arise during the genetic counseling session. Many deaf individuals use text messaging for communicating with family and friends.

Asking About a Family History of Deafness

Genetic counselors who want to take down a family history of deafness from a deaf client will usually need to explain carefully why this is necessary. Some deaf clients are sensitive to being asked about their family, given that, in the past, this information was used against them in the name of eugenic practices. A suspicion about this still remains (Middleton et al. 2010a). However, once the deaf client is reassured as to why it is important to ask about his or her family history of deafness, many individuals are interested in describing their family to, and sharing family stories with, the genetic counselor.

An Inappropriate Focus on Deafness

Iezzoni et al. (2004) interviewed deaf and hard-of-hearing people on their views about the healthcare system. They reported that "respondents wondered why physicians repeatedly question them about what caused their deafness when hearing is irrelevant to their current health concerns" (Iezzoni et al. 2004, 358).

> Research has shown that deaf clients are sometimes fed up that they are repeatedly asked about their deafness and also about deafness in their family. This is particularly important for deaf clients who have been referred for genetic counseling to discuss an issue unrelated to deafness.

Genetic counselors should be respectful of the fact that many deaf people do not see their deafness as a medical problem that needs to be explored.

Visual Aids

Deaf and hard-of-hearing people tend to be very "visual" and respond well to the use of diagrams, animations, and hand signals (e.g., one hand to indicate a recessive gene and another to indicate a dominant gene). Incorporating visual aids into a consultation is vitally important for deaf clients.

Emotional Issues to Consider in a Consultation

Deafness can be very disabling to a person, irrespective of his or her positive attitude or perspective of deafness. Most deaf and hard-of-hearing people have experienced "audism," a form of discrimination based on an individual's ability to hear or behave like someone who hears (Bauman 2004), at some point in their lives, and many experience this bias on a daily basis. It is known that deaf people generally have a higher risk than hearing people of having mental health issues (Department of Health 2005), likely as a result of audism, and therefore allowance must be made within any consultation for emotional fragility. The genetic counselor must not be surprised if there are sometimes frustration and seemingly overactive emotional responses.

> It is likely that the deaf client will have previous negative experiences of communicating with health professionals, and this may mean that he or she is defensive or aggressive in anticipation of poor service again. It can also help to use basic counseling skills, such as acknowledging openly some of the obvious difficulties.

For example, by saying things like "I can see you are really frustrated; however, I'm going to try really hard to understand what is going on for you" or "I can understand that you are fed up with health professionals; help me to learn what I need to do to help you."

Post-Clinic Letters

Genetic counselors will need to adapt the standard post-clinic letter for deaf and hard-of-hearing clients. This needs to be written in Plain English for deaf people so that when it is read they can easily translate it into sign language. Alternatively, information delivered directly in sign language and provided electronically would be best practice for Deaf clients (although not appropriate for hard-of-hearing non–sign language users). An online search will easily locate specialist companies that can translate client letters from standard written English into Plain English for Deaf people, as well as into sign language on DVD. Such work can often be completed within 24 hours. Alternatively, online resources of genetic information delivered in sign language can be accessed via the Internet. For example, the University of Manchester has produced video in BSL that describes different inheritance patterns and also provides information about genetic deafness. This can be viewed at http://sites.mhs.manchester.ac.uk/what-is-genetic-counselling/. By 2013, the website DeafMD.org will have cancer genetic information available in ASL (see Box 1.3).

Box 1.3 Case Study 3: Genetic counseling Delivered Visually

Roberto and his wife Maria attend a genetic counseling consultation in London. They are both profoundly deaf, and their first language is British Sign Language (BSL). Their genetic counselor, Alison, is not familiar with BSL and so established prior to the session that the couple prefers a BSL/English interpreter. Alison booked a local freelance worker who is a full member of the National Registers of Communication Professionals working with Deaf and Deafblind People (NRCPD) (she checked through the Signature website), thereby ensuring that a qualified and trained professional would provide interpreting for the session. Alison has already had a long chat with the interpreter on the phone to discuss the sorts of genetic terminology she will be describing in the consultation and how she plans to structure the session. They have discussed how the interpreter plans to sign particular concepts, such as "dominant inheritance" and "gene alteration." Alison has also given the interpreter a basic biology lesson on what DNA is, as well as what is meant by "gene," "chromosome," and "genome." In addition, she has sent some written information and drawings in a post to the interpreter. Alison has also provided information about the room they will using and how the light is positioned, and has already given some thought to appropriate seating arrangements. In the consultation, Roberto and Maria ask for information about the chances of having deaf children. It is clear to Alison that there is a dominantly inherited, genetic deafness on Roberto's side of the family and an environmental cause to Maria's deafness. Alison first defines the terms she is going to use—"genome," "chromosome," "gene," and "DNA"—and shows the couple pictures of these using a library metaphor—the DNA represents the words in a book, each individual book represents a gene, each shelf of books represents a chromosome, and a set of shelves represents a genome. She checks that the couple are following her and asks several times for them to give feedback on what she is saying, so that she can check their understanding. When Alison describes dominant inheritance, she draws on a piece of paper, being careful to not talk at the same time so that the couple can watch her draw. When they look up she describes what she has drawn. To reinforce the points she is making, she also describes dominant inheritance using her two hands to represent two genes; she moves her hands to indicate one gene being passed on and the other not. The interpreter also uses the same nomenclature. Alison asks Roberto and Maria to summarize their understanding of the genetic terminology and also asks them to draw out the inheritance pattern. At the end of the consultation, Alison gives the couple a DVD containing a National Sign Language (NSL) version of the department leaflet "What Is Dominant Inheritance?" so that they have a signed record of the information.

Comment

Alison has used four different visual methods to relay information—pre-printed pictures, live drawing, hand signals, and a DVD summary. This has all been delivered in sign language, with several opportunities to repeat and rephrase the different concepts. The couple's understanding has also been checked throughout the consultation. In England, Wales, and Northern Ireland a list of NRCPD-registered interpreters can be found at www.signature.org.uk. In the United States, a list of certified interpreters can be found through www.rid.org.

Case study taken from Middleton (2009b).

SUMMARY

This chapter has offered an insight into those issues of relevance and importance to deaf and hard-of-hearing people and described the sorts of preparation that genetic professionals should make for consultations involving this client group.

- Deafness can be perceived in different ways, and this can have an impact on how a consultation should be delivered.
- The different forms of communication require counselors to choose the most appropriate interpreters for each individual client.
- The unique historical context of eugenics and deafness, and its potential impact on modern-day consultation, is of particular significance to genetic counseling for deaf people.
- Much work needs to be done before and during a consultation to meet the communication needs of the deaf client.

At present, deaf and hard-of-hearing clients rarely access genetic counseling services, not due to disinterest but due to barriers that prevent access. Once these access issues are addressed—and numerous research studies across the world are providing the evidence to help unravel these—then more deaf and hard-of-hearing clients will seek genetic counseling. It is, therefore, vital that genetic professionals are adequately prepared to work sensitively with this client group.

REFERENCES

Baldwin, E. E., Boudreault, P., Fox, M., Sinsheimer, J. S., & Palmer. C. G. S. (2011). Effect of pre-test genetic counseling for deaf adults on knowledge of genetic testing. *Journal of Genetic Counseling, 19,* 161–173.

Barnett, S. (2002). Communication with deaf and hard of hearing people: a guide for medical education. *Academic Medicine, 77*(7): 694–700.

Bauman, H-D. L. (2004). Audism: exploring the metaphysics of oppression. *Journal of Deaf Studies and Deaf Education, 9*(2): 239–246.

Boudreault, P., Baldwin, E. E., Fox, M., Dutton, L., Tullis, L., Linden, J., et al. (2010). Deaf adults' reasons for genetic testing depend on cultural affiliation: results from a prospective, longitudinal genetic counseling and testing study. *Journal of Deaf Studies and Deaf Education, 15:*209–227.

British Deaf Association. (2005). *Factsheet on using a sign language interpreter.* London: British Deaf Association. www.bda.org.uk

Department of Health. (2005). *Mental health and deafness: towards equity and access Best practice guidelines.* Available at: http://www.dh.gov.uk/en/Publicationsandstatistics/Publications/PublicationsPolicyAndGuidance/DH_4103995. (Accessed April 7, 2012).

Dolnick, E. (1993). Deafness as culture. *The Atlantic Monthly, 272*(3): 37–53.

Dye, M., & Kyle, J. (2001). *Deaf people in the community: health and disability.* Bristol: Deaf Studies Trust.

Enns, E. E., Boudreault, P., & Palmer, C. G. S. (2010). Examining the relationship between genetic counselors' attitudes toward deaf people and the genetic counseling session. *Journal of Genetic Counseling, 19*: 161–173.

Erting, C. (1994). *Deafness, communication, social identity: ethnography in a pre-school for deaf children.* Burtonsville, MD: Linstock Press.

Fischer, S. D., & van der Hulst, H. (2003). Sign language structures. In M Marschark & P. E. Spencer (Eds.), *Oxford Handbook of Deaf Studies, Language, and Education.* New York: Oxford University Press. 319–331

Grundfast, K. M., & Rosen, J. (1992). Ethical and cultural considerations in research on hereditary deafness. *Otolaryngologic Clinics of North America, 25*(5): 973–978.

Harmer, L. M. (1999). Health care delivery and deaf people: practice, problems, and recommendations for change. *Journal of Deaf Studies and Deaf Education, 4*(2): 73–110.

Hoffmeister, R. (1985). Families with deaf parents: a functional perspective. In K. Thurman (Ed.), *Children of handicapped parents: research and clinical perspective* (pp. 111–130). Orlando, FL: Academic Press.

Iezzoni, L. I., O'Day, B. L., Killeen, M., & Harker, H. (2004). Communicating about health care: observations from persons who are deaf or hard of hearing. *Annals of Internal Medicine, 140*: 356–362.

Israel, J., &Arnos, K . (1995). *Genetic evaluation and counseling strategies: the genetic services center experience. An introduction to deafness: a manual for genetic counselors* (pp. 181–208). Washington DC: Genetic Services Center, Gallaudet University.

Ladd, P. (2003). *Understanding Deaf culture: in search of Deafhood.* Clevedon, UK: Multilingual Matters.

Martinez, A., Linden, J., Schimmenti, L. A., & Palmer, C. G. S. (2003). Attitudes of the broader hearing, deaf, and hard-of-hearing community toward genetic testing for deafness. *Genetics in Medicine, 5:*106–112.

Meadow, K. P. (1980). *Deafness and child development.* Berkeley: University of California Press.

Middleton, A. (2009a). General themes to consider when working with deaf and hard of hearing clients. In A. Middleton (Ed.), *Working with deaf people—a handbook for health professionals* (pp. 29–70). Cambridge: Cambridge University Press.

Middleton, A. (2009b). Specialist issues relevant to working with d/Deaf clients. In A. Middleton (Ed.), *Working with deaf people—a handbook for health professionals (pp. 84–128).* Cambridge: Cambridge University Press.

Middleton, A., Hewison, J., & Mueller, R. F. (1998). Attitudes of deaf adults toward genetic testing for hereditary deafness. *American Journal Human Genetics, 63:* 1175–1180.

Middleton, A., Hewison, J., & Mueller, R. F. (2001). Prenatal diagnosis for inherited deafness – what is the potential demand? *Journal of Genetic Counseling, 10*(2): 121–131.

Middleton, A., Emery, S. D., & Turner, G. H. (2010a). Views, knowledge and beliefs about genetics and genetic counselling amongst people with deafness. *Sign Language Studies, 10*(2): 170–196.

Middleton, A., Turner, G., Bitner-Glindzicz, M., Lewis, P., Richards, M., Clarke, A., et al. (2010b). Preferences for communication in clinic from deaf people: a cross-sectional study. *Journal of Evaluation in Clinical Practice, 16*(4): 811–817.

Morton, C., &Nance, W. (2006). Newborn hearing screening—a silent revolution. *New England Journal of Medicine, 354:* 2151–2164.

Nance, W., Liu, X., Pandya, A., (2000). Relation between choice of partner and high frequency of connexin 26 deafness. *Lancet, 356:* 500–501.

Padden, C., &Humphries, T. (2005). *Inside Deaf culture.* London: Harvard University Press.

Prosser, S., &Martini, A. (2007).Understanding the phenotype: basic concepts in audiology. Genes, hearing and deafness. In A. Martini, D. Stephens, & A. P. Read (Eds.), *From molecular biology to clinical practice* (pp. 19–38). London: Informa Healthcare.

Reeves, D., & Kokoruwe, B. (2005). Communication and communication support in Primary care: a survey of deaf patients. *Audiological Medicine, 3:* 95–107.

RNID (2004). *A simple cure.* London: Royal National Institute for Deaf People.

Schein, J. D. (1989). *Family life: at home among strangers* (pp. 106–134). Washington, DC: Gallaudet University Press.

Schuchman, J. (2004). Deafness and eugenics in the Nazi era. Genetics. In J. V. V. Cleve (Ed.), *Disability and deafness.* Washington DC: Gallaudet University Press.p72–78.

Smith, R., & Van Camp. G., (2010, 02/12/08). *Deafness and hereditary hearing loss overview.* Available from http://www.ncbi.nlm.nih.gov. (Accessed on March 24, 2010.)

Steinberg, A. G., Barnett, S., Meador, H., El, Wiggins, E, A., Zazove, P,. (2006). Health care system accessibility: experiences and perceptions of deaf people. *Journal of General Internal Medicine, 21:* 260–266.

Stephens, D., & Danermark, B. (2005). The international classification of functioning, disability and health as a conceptual framework for the impact of genetic hearing impairment. In D. Stephens & L. Jones (Eds.), *The impact of genetic hearing impairment* (pp. 54–67). London: Whurr.

Withrow, K. A., Tracy, K. A., Burton, S. K., Norris, V. S., Maes, H. H., Arnos, K. S., et al. (2009). Provision of genetic services for hearing loss: Results from a national survey and comparison to insights obtained from previous focus group discussions. *Journal of Genetic Counseling, 18:*618–621.

2 Communicating with Clients Who Are Visually Impaired

Georgina Hall and Alison Clarke

Communicate unto the other person that which you would want him to communicate unto you, if your positions were reversed.
—Aaron Goldman

Genetic services for families with inherited eye conditions are expanding rapidly. This has been driven by the increasing knowledge of the genetic basis of visual impairment (VI) and the consequent improvements in diagnostic tools, including genetic testing.

In the United Kingdom, the National Health Service (NHS) has been widely criticized for its failure to meet the communication needs of partially sighted and blind people, recently highlighted by the British support group, Royal National Institute of Blind People (RNIB)'s Losing Patients Campaign (www.rnib.org.uk/losingpatients) and Lost for Words (2010). A U.K. survey of 600 blind and partially sighted people found that 72% could not read the health information that they were provided (Sibley 2009). More recently, RNIB Scotland reported that although 95% of people had a preferred reading format, only 10% of all communications from health services were provided in a chosen format. This study reported that people did not complain when information was received in an inappropriate format; they did, however, say they felt a loss of autonomy and privacy in accessing information, a lack of general understanding of their additional needs, and the need to frequently rely on others (Thurston 2010).

A primary goal of genetic counseling is the provision of information (Clarke 1997). Genetic information is sometimes complex and difficult for the lay person to understand. Individuals may need to absorb a lot of new information that is highly technical and abstract. Traditionally, genetic service providers have used diagrams to explain inheritance patterns and summary letters or written leaflets to reinforce explanations provided in clinic. These communication tools are not appropriate for client with VI, and a recent audit in Manchester, United Kingdom, confirmed that communication tools in genetic eye services do not meet client needs (personal communication Hall and Clarke 2008).

This chapter describes the impact of visual impairment and the needs of clients attending genetic eye clinics. We highlight the additional communication provision required by clients, including alternate appointment formats, availability of alternate counseling aids, and the importance of recording communication needs and providing written information in different formats (see Box 2.1).

Box 2.1 Case Study 1

Ian, aged 29, requested referral to the genetic eye clinic. Ian's vision had begun deteriorating in his teens and, as a result, he had dropped out of school. Over the years, he had seen a number of different eye doctors in his local hospital, and he had been given several different names for his condition, including rod-cone dystrophy and retinitis pigmentosa. There had been no previous family history of eye problems, apart from a grandparent with glaucoma. Ian had been told there was no cure for his eye condition and had been discharged from the eye specialists.

Ian was currently unemployed. He had spent a number of years feeling very angry about his vision problem; he became very isolated and had lost confidence in going out. He had recently heard a news article about new treatments for retinitis pigmentosa and had requested an appointment in the eye clinic. His general practitioner referred him to the genetic eye clinic.

In preparation for the clinic, the genetic counselor was aware of the significant emotional and psychosocial impact that the visual impairment (VI) may be having on Ian and planned to take a thorough psychosocial history. In addition, the genetic counselor was aware of the complex genetic information around the diagnosis, and of the terminology and different possible inheritance patterns for the genes that might be involved in his condition. Ian met both the consultant ophthalmologist and the genetic counselor. He was examined and a diagnosis of retinal dystrophy was confirmed. Ian was told there was no cure for the condition and that his vision would continue to deteriorate.

Using adapted communication tools, the genetic counselor reviewed the possible inheritance patterns of retinal dystrophy, and a blood test was taken for future genetic testing. The genetic counselor also listened carefully to Ian's experiences and felt that he was depressed and isolated. He was registered as severely sight impaired, and the genetic counselor agreed to contact the VI team at the hospital to request further

(Continued)

Box 2.1 (Continued)

support as well as referring Ian for further counseling and practical and emotional support from local VI support groups.

A year later, Ian returned to the genetic eye clinic. He was still unemployed, but he was taking a computer course and hoped to use his new computer skills in future work. He had joined a blind football team and had a network of friends. Genetic testing had revealed a change in an X-linked RP gene. The genetic counselor could review this inheritance pattern and discuss the risks to future children and the possible implications for his wider family.

BACKGROUND

Definitions of Visual Impairment

"Vision impairment" is an umbrella term for any level of reduced vision and is often used alongside the terms "blind" and "partially sighted."

> Choosing the best terminology with clients in the clinic is important; the term "blind" can be emotive and often carries the misconception of complete lack of vision. It may be advisable to avoid this term in the clinic, particularly until the term and its meaning have been explained. The terms most widely accepted include "partially sighted," "vision impairment," and "sight loss."

Visual impairment or low vision may be defined as a severe reduction in vision that cannot be corrected with standard glasses or contact lenses and that reduces a person's ability to function at certain or all tasks. Legally, people with VI fall into two groups: "partial sight impairment" and "severe sight impairment" (blind). Severe sight impairment ("legally blind") is measured by visual acuity (reading letters down a chart) and visual fields. Clients are registered as severely sight impaired if their best corrected vision is 20/200 or less or if their visual field is no greater than 20 degrees (i.e., peripheral vision is reduced to "tunnel" vision). It must be remembered that many "blind" clients retain some level of vision that remains important to them in everyday life.

Since the mid-1930s, there has been a national system in the United Kingdom for registering people who are partially sighted or blind, currently known as the Certificate of Vision Impairment (CVI, formally known as the BD8) (Bunce et al. 2010). Registration is voluntary and has a dual aim of coordinating support services and collecting epidemiology data. In the United States, a similar system of "legally blind" registration provides access to state provision of services and tax exemption.

The RNIB is the largest support group in the United Kingdom for blind and partially signed people. The RNIB estimates that sight loss affects around two million people in the United Kingdom (www.rnib.org.uk/statistics). The vast majority are older people, but an estimated 80,000 working-age adults and 25,000 children in the United Kingdom are affected by sight problems, with an approximate incidence of 1 in 136. The American Foundation for the Blind (AFB), the national support organization in the United States, reports more than 25 million people with vision loss in that country.

In the United Kingdom, the registration system records the number of people who are blind or partially sighted. The number of people eligible for registration is rising, and this trend is expected to continue due to an ageing population and increased survival rates of babies with complex inherited conditions including sight loss (Binns 2009; Moore & Burton 2008; NHS 2008). In addition, around 28% of those registered have an additional disability (NHS 2008).

By far the leading cause of VI is age-related macular dystrophy (AMD), accounting for 58% of severe sight impaired and 57% of partial sight impaired registration in 2007–8 (Bunce et al. 2010). The next most frequent causes are glaucoma, diabetic retinopathy, and hereditary retinal disorders. It is estimated that hereditary retinal conditions account for 15% of VI in working-age adults (Moore & Burton 2008). The most common retinal dystrophy is retinitis pigmentosa, affecting 1 in 3,500 individuals in the United States and Europe (Black 2002). As the prevalence of treatable conditions (such as retinopathy of prematurity) decreases, the proportion of untreatable, genetic causes of VI will increase.

Legal and Ethical Framework

The United Nations (UN) convention on the Rights of Persons with Disabilities (ratified 2007) describes the fundamental rights of disabled people for full and equal freedoms, including independent living, full inclusion in the community, and access to health, education, employment, and leisure. In the United Kingdom, the Disability Discrimination Act (1995) and the Disability and Equality Act (2010) clarify the legal obligation to meet the needs of blind and partially sighted clients. These also cover employment and access to services.

In the United States, "The Americans with Disabilities Act of 1990 (ADA) is a federal civil rights law that prohibits discrimination against individuals with disabilities in everyday activities, including medical services. Section 504 of the Rehabilitation Act of 1973 (Section 504) is a civil rights law that prohibits discrimination against individuals with disabilities on the basis of their disability in programs or activities that receive federal financial assistance, including health programs and services. These statutes require medical care providers to make their services available in an accessible manner" (http://www.ada.gov/medcare_mobility_ta/medcare_ta.htm).

These imperatives have direct relevance to standard genetic counseling practice. For example, sending letters in regular small print to a person with a visual disability is an infringement of his or her human rights, taking away his or her autonomy to access written information and his or her privacy.

Inherited Eye Conditions

Inherited eye conditions are a highly heterogeneous group of conditions in terms of their genetic basis, age of onset, and association with other health problems. They range from congenital disorders, such as microphthalmia, to glaucoma development and cataracts. Many affect only vision, and morbidity is directly related to loss of sight. However, a significant number may present alongside other developmental abnormalities—for example, about 50% of clients with microphthalmia have learning difficulties. Another large group of disorders is the inherited retinal dystrophies, which may present at birth (e.g., Leber congenital amaurosis, achromatopsia), during early childhood (e.g., X-linked retinitis pigmentosa), or even in adult life (e.g., Sorsby macular dystrophy). For a full description of the range of inherited eye conditions, see Black (2002).

Despite improving characterizations and burgeoning ophthalmic imaging techniques, genetic eye conditions are rare, and experience within general ophthalmology clinics remains limited. Thus, specialist services are important for accurate diagnosis as a prerequisite for genetic counseling—for example, in a 6-month audit in 2007, the multidisciplinary genetic eye clinics in Manchester recorded that 30% of families received a new diagnosis after attending the specialist clinic and a further 15% had their diagnosis changed. Experience shows that many individuals receive different diagnostic opinions and can spend many years in search of a diagnosis, all of which must underpin the counseling process.

The specific challenges relating to genetic counseling for inherited eye conditions include accurate diagnosis in the face of extreme genetic heterogeneity (e.g., retinitis pigmentosa may involve up to 200 different genes—see Retnet (2010) for a current list of genes and loci). Ophthalmic examination alone is often unable to distinguish one type from another, so that accurate family history within the context of genetic counseling is very important.

As a result, assessing the inheritance pattern can be difficult in many individuals even once a specific clinical diagnosis has been made. With the rapid advances in genetic testing, it is highly likely that next-generation or massively parallel sequencing will be very important in accurate diagnosis in many of these heterogeneous groups of eye conditions (Koenekoop, Lopez, Den Hollander, Allikmets, & Cremers 2007).

As diagnosis and potential for treatments become available, the client demand for testing and genetic counseling for information around genetic risk increases. Within the genetic service, protocols are in place for dealing with predictive testing and presymptomatic genetic diagnosis. Within the ophthalmic setting, the potential impact of presymptomatic diagnosis, either through genetic testing or by ocular examination, has not been given the same consideration. The benefits of presymptomatic testing may be clear if treatment is available to either delay or prevent the development of disease pathology. The advantages are less clear if testing does not have therapeutic implications and only provides information. A positive gene test or an ocular examination revealing early signs of disease in a currently asymptomatic individual would indicate that he or she is likely to develop a visual problem but may provide limited information about the age of onset or the severity of visual loss. One of the major reasons individuals consider having a presymptomatic test is to provide certainty, but testing may not provide the degree of certainty being sought. Possible benefits of presymptomatic testing for inherited eye disease include the ability to make informed decisions regarding issues such as employment and child bearing. In addition, the time prior to the onset of visual problems may be used for preparation in both a practical and emotional sense for future VI.

Psychosocial Impact of Visual Impairment

Unlike the Deaf community, families and clients with low vision perceive VI as a disability. The degree to which people come to terms with and accept their sight loss is highly variable.

Many people with VI adapt highly successfully and, with support and access to visual aids, computers, and technology, are able to access many levels of employment, leisure activities, and independent living. However, genetic counselors are often meeting clients when they are newly diagnosed, and this is a critical time for offering support and signposting to relevant support services.

Visual impairment has a significant impact on an individual's life, affecting many aspect of daily living including shopping, reading, outdoor mobility, and leisure pursuits (Lamoureux et al. 2004). It is well described that individuals with VI have high rates of depression, particularly in the older population. Evans et al. (2007) found the prevalence of depression is at least twice as high in older adults with VI. Nyman et al. (2010) reviewed the literature on the psychosocial impact of vision loss in working-age adults and found that adults with VI have significantly higher levels of mental health issues and lower levels of social functioning and quality of life. A recent survey found that only 34% of blind and partially sighted people are employed, compared to 75% of the population over all (Clements & Douglas 2009). In addition, 24% of blind and partially sighted people of working age have no qualifications, compared to 15% of the general population (Pey 2007). This evidence demonstrates that many VI clients are disadvantaged, with reduced access to education and employment.

> Many genetic forms of adult-onset VI cause a progressive deterioration in vision. Clients go through repeated periods of vision loss and readjustment, requiring ongoing support. The process of visual loss has been likened to a grief reaction, requiring a process of adjustment and adaptation. Many individuals need support, in the form of both emotional support and practical guidance, to help them regain confidence and learn new skills. Periods of denial are common, and many people feel very reluctant to give up aspects of their life and independence, such as driving. Loneliness and isolation is a common problem as people lose confidence in their ability to go out and feel less able to participate in society.

Although vision itself may deteriorate slowly, key events may evoke further periods of grief and adaptation (e.g., when driving is no longer possible, when employment is threatened). It can be particularly difficult when the individual had adapted and was living successfully with a particular level of vision and has to face a period of change. In this way, genetic counselors should not assume that a person with a long-standing diagnosis of VI is coping when they attend a genetic eye clinic.

Practical support is also very important. Genetic counselors should ensure that families have access to information and support from a range of services, including low vision aid clinics, eye clinic liaison officers, social services, education support services, employment support services, and regional and local charities.

Sight Loss and Communication

The methods of communication used by VI people may vary depending on whether vision loss has been "acquired" (come on later in life) or present since birth. For example, individuals born blind are more likely to have learned Braille at school than are those who have lost their vision later in life. In addition, clients with syndromic blindness may have additional communication needs relating, for example, to learning difficulties. In some cases, clients may have dual sensory impairment involving both hearing and vision, and this small group of clients has very special needs.

The spectrum of sight loss among inherited eye conditions is very broad. Conditions that affect central vision (including cone dystrophy, macular dystrophy) will reduce an individual's use of macular vision, including detail perception (recognizing faces, reading or watching television), sight in well-lit conditions, and reduced color perception. Conditions affecting particularly the peripheral vision (retinal dystrophy, primary open-angle glaucoma) will present with reduced night vision, difficulty in navigation, and an awareness of objects appearing suddenly at the side. In the severe form, this is called tunnel vision. Many conditions (cone-rod dystrophy, cataract) affect aspects of both the central and peripheral vision. Clients may suffer from photophobia (difficulty in bright lights) or "night blindness" (difficulty in dimly lit conditions and particularly adjusting when moving from light to dark areas).

PREPARING FOR THE CONSULTATION

Many hospitals continue to send written appointments in small print to clients with VI. In their survey, Sibley (2009) found that one-fifth of blind and partially sighted respondents said they had missed an appointment due to information being sent in a format they could not read themselves.

This is clearly a critical problem from the client's perspective in accessing potentially important healthcare interventions, as well as for the service providers and missed appointments. Barriers to provision of accessible appointments include the appointment database systems themselves, staff training, and resources. At the very least, appointment letters should comply with clear-print guidelines, and more information is given about this later (RNIB 2002). To manage this effectively, hospital systems should include the capability to record client preference and provide appointment notification in larger print or by telephone or e-mail.

Key points to remember include:

- Blind and partially sighted people report missing appointments due to inaccessible letters.
- Letters should comply with clear-print guidelines.
- Every effort should be made to provide appointments in formats required by clients including large print, telephone calls, or e-mail.

Practical Considerations in the Genetic Clinic

People with VI attending genetic clinics will require varying levels of practical support during the consultations. The following lists some of the considerations that should be taken into account by the genetic counselor:

- Visually impaired clients may bring a support person to help navigate to the outpatient department. This support person may be a friend or family member, or they may be a volunteer support person provided through a charity, for example. It is important to inquire whether the client wants the support person with them in clinic. If not, the genetic counselor will need to guide the client into clinic (see below).
- Some VI clients navigate with the aid of a guide dog or a white cane. In tight settings, such as an outpatient waiting room, it can be helpful to offer to guide the person into the clinic room.

Box 2.2 Case Study 2

George, aged 61, was referred to the ophthalmic genetic clinic by the ophthalmologist at his local hospital. He had been experiencing deteriorating vision for a couple of years and was finding it increasingly difficult to get out and about and to live independently. The referral letter indicated that George attended the ophthalmology clinic with his grandson and, when George arrived for his genetic eye clinic appointment, it was initially assumed that the young man accompanying him was his grandchild. However, on further inquiry, the genetic counsellor established that the young man was actually George's neighbor's son, a college student, who helped George with shopping, reading the mail, and getting to appointments, in exchange for payment to help supplement his limited finances. Although George relied on this assistance and valued it a great deal, he disliked asking for help from a neighbor and found his loss of independence very difficult to accept. In addition, his young helper was about to go off to the university, leaving George anxious about how he would cope.

The genetic counselor was able to discuss various sources of help and support with George, including registration as being severely visually impaired and referral to his local social service department and their visual impairment team. As a consequence, George was able to access mobility training and advice on various pieces of equipment to help him carry out daily activities like reading the mail with the aid of a closed circuit (CCTV). This enabled George to continue living independently, and he also felt his self-esteem and quality of life improved considerably.

- When offering to guide a VI client, it is most helpful to allow him or her to take the back of your arm and walk to the side, just ahead of the person. Be aware of obstacles and tell him or her when you have reached the chair, so that he or she can navigate to a seated position.
- Adapting the room to help the vision of a client can be helpful. Some clients may like a well lit room whereas others might have better vision in dimmer lighting.
- Remember that VI clients may not be aware of other people in the room (e.g., doctors observing a clinic), and it is important to introduce and make them aware of who is present and who is speaking. See Box 2.2.

COMMUNICATION IN THE CONSULTATION

Counseling Tools

Because of the complex nature of material conveyed during genetic outpatient clinic consultations, a number of tools are used to aid understanding. These include the use of diagrams and pictorial representations of inheritance patterns and chromosomes.

Recent evidence supports the use of "personalized" diagrams in helping families put the scientific information into the context of their family (Gale, Pasalosdos-Sanchez, Kerzin-Storrar, Hall, & Macleod 2010). However, clients with VI are disadvantaged because these traditional tools are not accessible.

There are a number of options for adapting pictures and diagrams for use with visually impaired clients. First, it can be very useful to have a thick black marker. Many clients can access a drawing if it is bold and large, and this is a very easy way to use drawing to communicate with visually impaired clients. Some genetic clinics have developed enlarged print diagrams, but computers can also be a useful tool in helping with accessibility of information.

Computer assistive technology was recently trialed in genetic eye clinics in Manchester. Many clients use magnifiers for reading (Douglas, Corcoran, & Pavey 2006).

Closed circuit television (CCTV) cameras allow the genetic counselor to enlarge diagrams from standard counseling aids onto a big screen. Computer software such as Zoomtext or Supernova allows the magnification of electronic images, such as a PDF version of Mendelian inheritance diagrams. A large computer screen on an extendable arm allows the screen to be drawn nearer to the client. The additional advantage of these magnifying techniques is the ability to vary not only the size of the diagram but also its color and background, for example, using a light image on a dark background (inverse brightness). These tools allow the genetic counselor to find the best image to suit each individual.

The computer screen can also be useful when counseling a number of family members, with the enlarged diagrams simultaneously accessible for the sighted members seated across the room (see Box 2.3).

Box 2.3 Case Study 3

Malcolm attended a genetic clinic with his wife Sarah, to discuss his diagnosis of Stargardt's macular dystrophy. Despite attending the genetic clinic on a few occasions, Malcolm and Sarah wanted to review the inheritance of Stargardt's, and they were hoping to start a family. The genetic counselor was careful not to assume Malcolm's level of vision; he was able to navigate around the clinic without any difficulty, and he kept good eye contact when speaking to the genetic counselor. During the consultation, the genetic counselor inquired about Malcolm's vision, asking about the things he found difficult, such as reading and recognizing faces.

(Continued)

Box 2.3 (Continued)

Malcolm confirmed that he had difficulty reading, and so the genetic counselor asked if he would mind her using the computer diagrams to help with the discussion. The genetic counselor was able to move the computer screen so that it was close to Malcolm. She used a number of different magnifications and inverted the brightness until Malcolm was happy that he could see the images on the screen. Using the computer screen, Sarah was also able to have a good view of the images while sitting beside Malcolm, back from the desk.

Malcolm and Sarah felt fully involved with the discussion and, despite having had the explanation before, they reported a much greater understanding of the genes and inheritance pattern using the computer diagrams. They were reassured by the low risk to future children. The genetic counselor asked how they would like their summary letter. Malcolm said that he used a computer at home with magnification and speech software and provided his e-mail address. They also requested a printed copy for Sarah and their records. The genetic counselor gave them a CD-ROM with an audio file describing autosomal recessive inheritance.

Tactile Diagrams

Clients with severe VI will not be able to access all visual diagrams. Tactile diagrams may therefore be necessary. Working with the RNIB tactile diagram center and a focus group of clients, optimal tactile inheritance diagrams were designed for the genetic eye clinic (Clarke, Hall, Turgut, Trump, & Black 2010). Diagrams that seem visually simple can be complicated and confusing when navigated by touch. Symbols easily distinguished visually, such as squares and circles, are not as easy to distinguish on a tactile diagram. Therefore, designing a tactile diagram needs consultation with a professional team, such as that provided by the RNIB.

Using a tactile diagram with visually impaired client also requires practice. Clients like to have independent use of the diagram. Each diagram has a navigation point to tell the user how the page should be oriented. Once the user is holding the page, he or she may want to explore the image before the genetic counselor describes the diagram. The genetic counselor can then guide the client through the image (e.g., "On the top left hand side, you will feel a pair of genes …"). It is helpful to break down the explanation into different images, as complex diagrams with lots of lines and arrows can be very difficult to follow.

Key points to remember include:

• Always have a thick black marker available because many clients with VI will be able to access a drawing when it is produced in large black print.

- Diagrams can be simplified and enlarged for use in genetic eye clinics.
- Specialist clinics may consider investing in assistive technology to help the accessibility of counseling aids. These may include CCTV magnifiers or magnification software on computer screens.
- Tactile diagrams can be very useful, but preparation and experience is needed to develop and use them effectively.
- Experience shows that clients appreciate these adaptations to communication aids in clinic.

Print Information

Given the variation of VI, blind and partially sighted people will have varying needs in terms of accessing information. Different people will have different preferences, and therefore a range of formats must be available (McBride 2000). Evidence from the United Kingdom has shown that the majority of blind and partially sighted people are not able to access the written health information they receive (Sibley 2009).

Research studies funded by lay organizations representing visually impaired individuals have shown that people with VI do not tend to complain when information is received in the wrong format, even when they know they have a right to receive information in alternate formats (Sibley 2009; Thurston 2010).

A lack of requests from clients does not indicate a lack of need. Sibley (2009) expresses the concern that clients with VI not asking for information in accessible formats may be reinforcing healthcare professionals' belief that they do not want it. Healthcare providers must be more proactive in offering information in a variety of formats.

It is difficult to get accurate information about the demand for different formats. Network 1000 (Douglas, Corcoran, & Pavey, 2006), a consultation group of approximately 1,000 visually impaired people, provides survey and statistical data on the changing needs of people with VI. This random sample did not reflect exactly the same proportion of blind versus partially sighted people in the United Kingdom population, but, as a random sample, it does give some helpful indications of the range of communication needs. When questioned about their ability to read print, 18% could read ordinary newspaper print, 52% could read enlarged print, and 30% reported they could not read print without the aid of a magnifier. Five percent reported they read Braille, and the majority of these are individuals who have been visually impaired since childhood. The most popular method for reading was audio tapes (72%), and 44% described having someone to read to them. Individuals with visual impairment use different resources and have different preferences in accessing printed information.

The RNIB clear-print guidelines (RNIB 2002) are based on sound research findings and the RNIB's experience of the needs of visually impaired individuals. They highlight what factors need to be considered when designing and producing printed materials that take into account the needs of people with visual problems and make these materials accessible to a wider audience. These factors include font, type size, contrast, and layout (RNIB 2002).

It is easy to get print information converted into different formats, including Braille and audio files. The United Kingdom Association for Accessible Formats (UKAAF) represent individuals and organizations committed to providing information formats to improve the social inclusion of blind and partially sighted people. There are many organizations that offer transcription services, including the RNIB (http://www.rnib.org.uk/aboutus/contactdetails/nireland/nireading/Pages/accessiblemediani.aspx) and other private companies such as Pia (http://www.pia.co.uk). In the United States, the American Printing House for the Blind provides accessible formats and technology to support the accessibility of written information (http://www.aph.org).

It is our legal obligation to provide letters in an accessible format, if not the client's preferred format. To do this, we must first improve the practices of inquiring and recording the communication needs of our clients. Providing summary letters in large print is easy and cheap to achieve.

> It can be useful to have an example sheet of different font sizes in the clinic to help the client identify which size would be most accessible for him or her.

For severely sight impaired clients, any type of written information is inaccessible and alternatives such as audio files and Braille must be explored. Increasingly, blind and partially sighted people are using computer assistive technology, particularly those in younger generations. For these clients, an e-mailed letter can be accessed using computer voice software. In our experience, given these different formats, the actual numbers of clients requiring audio or Braille transcription is very small and not a cost burden to the department. The advantages to the clients outweigh this small cost over all.

Departments using standard leaflets should also explore alternate formats. Large print leaflets may be cheap to produce. Audio CDs are also cheap to produce once the original leaflet has been recorded as an audio file. Many leaflets include diagrams, and care should be taken when translating these. Transcription services have a lot of experience in producing materials for people with VI and are able to provide support in producing the best quality information.

SUMMARY

Key points to remember include:

- Clients tend not to ask for alternate formats as they assume they are not available. Lack of requests does not reflect a lack of need.

- A systematic approach is needed to request and record format preferences in client records. Use of an example sheet of different font sizes may aid in identifying preferences.
- All written information should aim to comply with clear-print guidelines.
- Where possible, written information should be offered in alternate formats:
  - Large print is cheap and easy to provide.
  - Letters may be e-mailed for clients to read with computer assistive software at home
  - A very small minority of clients may require transcription into audio or Braille.

Genetic counselors are accustomed to providing information in a way that is helpful and meaningful to clients. We are used to assessing client's understanding and being mindful of language barriers, culture issues, and learning and communication difficulties in the way we present information. Sight loss is very common, and clients with VI attending the genetic clinic for indications related or unrelated to visual loss (e.g., family history of cancer) may have additional communication needs. It is our ethical and legal duty to inquire about the accessibility of information in all clinics and to respond to communication needs. Evidence shows that we need to be more proactive in offering alternate formats because clients do not complain or demand accessible information even though it is their right to do so.

Most adaptations to written information are easily provided. All written materials should comply with clear-print guidelines, including appointment letters, summary letters, and leaflets. The cost of transcribing information into Braille or audio files is minimal, given the small number of clients for whom it is needed. Dedicated eye clinics may consider investing in assistive technology in clinic and tactile diagrams to make counseling aids accessible to all clients.

RESOURCES

American Foundation for the Blind (AFB): "AFB's priorities include broadening access to technology; elevating the quality of information and tools for the professionals who serve people with vision loss; and promoting independent and healthy living for people with vision loss by providing them and their families with relevant and timely resources. AFB's work in these areas is supported by its strong presence in Washington, D.C., ensuring the rights and interests of Americans with vision loss are represented in our nation's public policies."

Royal National Institute for the Blind (RNIB): This national U.K. charity provides many different resources for individuals with vision impairment in the United Kingdom; http://rnib.org.uk

National Blind Children's Society: The society supports blind and partially sighted children and their families in the United Kingdom; http://www.nbcs.org.uk/

Action for Blind People: This U.K. national charity provides practical support for visually impaired people. The organization has local offices around the United Kingdom; http://www.maculardisease.org/

Vision2020: This umbrella organization produces many publications relating to vision loss, including training, communication, and accessibility for patients with VI; http://www.vision2020uk.org.uk/

Vision Impairment Network for Counseling and Emotional Support (VINCE): http://www.vision2020uk.org.uk/news.asp?newsID=1301&section=

The American Printing House for the Blind: The world's largest provider of accessible educational and daily living products; http://www.aph.org

Individual support groups, such as:

RP Fighting Blindness: Information and support for families with retinal dystrophy http://www.rpfightingblindness.org.uk/

Macular Disease Society: http://www.maculardisease.org/

REFERENCES

Binns, A., Bunce, C., Dickinson, C., Harper, R., Tudor-Edwards, R., Woodhouse, M., et al. (2009). Low vision service outcomes: A systematic review. *Low visions service model evaluation project*. London: RNIB.

Black, G. (2002). *Genetics for ophthalmologists*. London: Remedica Publishing.

Bunce, C., Xing. W., et al. (2010). Causes of blind and partial sight certification in England and Wales: April 2007–March 2008. *Eye, 24*: 1692–1699.

Clarke, A. (1997). The process of genetic counselling. Beyond non-directiveness. In P. Harper & A. Clarke (Eds.), *Genetics society and clinical practice* (pp. 179–200). Oxford, UK: BIOS Scientific Publishers.

Clarke, A. R., Hall, G. E., Turgut, A., Trump, D., & Black, G. (2010). Tactile diagrams to improve communication with patients with severe visual impairment in the genetic counselling clinic. *European Journal of Human Genetics, 18*(Suppl. 1), 391.

Clements, B., & Douglas, G. (2009). *Network 1000 survey 1: Comparing the general and registered visually impaired populations executive summary report for the RNIB*. Accessed April 7, 2012 from http://www.rnib.org.uk/aboutus/research/reports/2010/network_1000_comparison_summary.doc

DDA (1995) Disability Discrimination Act. Accessed 24 Sep, 2012 from www.legislation.gov.uk

Disability and the Equality Act (2010). Accessed 24 Sep, 2012 from www.legislation.gov.uk

Douglas, G., Corcoran, C., & Pavey, S. (2006). *Network 1000: Opinions and circumstances of visually impaired people in Great Britain: Report based on over 1000 interviews*. Accessed April 7, 2012 from http://www.rnib.org.uk/Search/Pages/results.aspx?k=Network%201000:%20opinions%20and%20circumstances&s=All%20Sites

Evans, J. R., Fletcher, A. E., & Wormald, R. P. (2007). Depression and anxiety in visually impaired older people. *Ophthalmology, 114*(2), 283–288.

Gale, T., Pasalodos-Sanchez, S., Kerzin-Storrar, L., Hall, G., & Macleod, R. (2010). Explaining Mendelian inheritance in genetic consultations: An IPR study of counsellor and counselee experiences. *Journal of Genetic Counseling, 19*(1),55–67.

Hall, G., & Clarke, A. (2008). A regional multidisciplinary genetics ophthalmic clinic: An audit. *Personal communication.*

Koenekoop, R. K., Lopez, I., Den Hollander, A. I., Allikmets, R., & Cremers, F. P. (2007). Genetic testing for retinal dystrophies and dysfunctions: Benefits, dilemmas and solutions. *Clinical and Experimental Ophthalmology, 35*(5), 473–485.

Lamoureux, E. L., Hassell, J. B., & Keeffe, J. E. (2004). The determinants of participation in activities of dial living in people with impaired vision. *American Journal of Ophthalmology, 137*(2), 265–270.

McBride, S. (2000). *Patients talking: Hospital outpatient eye services—the sight impaired user's view.* London: RNIB. Accessed April 7, 2012 from www.rnib.org.uk

Moore, T., & Burton, H. (2008). *Genetic ophthalmology in focus. A needs assessment and review of specialist eye disorders.* Accessed April 7, 2012 from http://www.phgfoundation.org/file/4199

NHS. (2008). *People registered as blind and partially sighted 2008 report.* Accessed April 7, 2012 from http://signposting.ic.nhs.uk/?k=People+registered+as+blind+and+partially+sighted+2008+report

Nyman, S. R., Gosney, M. A., & Victor, C. R. (2010). Psychosocial impact of visual impairment in working-age adults. *British Journal of Ophthalmology, 94,* 1427–1431.

Pey, T. (2007). *Functionality and the needs of blind and partially sighted adults in the UK.* Accessed April 7, 2012 from www.guidedogs.org.uk

Retnet. (2010). *Summaries of genes and loci causing retinal diseases.* Accessed April 7, 2012 from http://www.sph.uth.tmc.edu/retnet/sum-dis.htm

Royal National Institute of Blind People (RNIB). (2002). *See it right. Clear print guidelines.* Accessed April 7, 2012 from www.rnib.org.uk

Royal National Institute of Blind People (RNIB). (2010). *Lost for words.* Accessed April 7, 2012 from http://www.rnib.org.uk/getinvolved/campaign/accesstoinformation/lostforwords/Pages/lost_for_words.aspx

Sibley, E. (2009). *Towards an inclusive health service: A research report into the availability of health information for blind and partially sighted people.* London: Dr. Foster Intelligence for RNIB.

Thurston, M. (2010). An inquiry into the emotional impact of sight loss and the counselling experiences and needs of blind and partially sighted people. *Counselling and Psychotherapy Research, 10*(1), 3–12.

3 Communicating with Clients Affected by Diverse Sex Development

Lih-Mei Liao and Margaret Simmonds

I like to listen. I have learned a great deal from listening carefully. Most people never listen.

—Ernest Hemingway

"Is it a boy or a girl?" This is by far the most likely first question ever asked about a human being. With prenatal testing becoming increasingly routine these days, the answer does not even have to wait until the baby arrives. But, what happens when the expected straightforward response to the question is not available? What do the reactions, often characterized by shock and confusion, tell us about some shared assumptions that we have about sex and gender? How are affected individuals and families to make sense of these situations, and how can clinicians discuss them in more helpful ways?

The stability of dimorphic sex categories in our society obscures the fact that all human embryos begin life with a common set of reproductive and genital structures. Sex differentiation typically begins at about 6 weeks of embryonic life, and a sex-undifferentiated fetus gradually assumes the anatomical structures and appearance of what we think of as male or female. The tissues that develop into the testes, penis, and scrotum in males are initially the same as those that develop into the ovaries, womb, vagina, clitoris, and labia in females.

A number of genetic conditions can disrupt regular embryonic sex differentiation and development, so that the outcomes may not clearly correspond to one of the two mutually exclusive physical sex categories recognized by most contemporary societies. That is to say, the usual markers of sex—karyotype, gonads, and genitalia—are not entirely male-typical or female-typical. The term "intersex" is often used to refer to these developmental outcomes (Hughes 2002). Further back in time, the term "hermaphroditism" prevailed (see Dreger et al. 2005). Numbers depend, of course, on inclusion criteria. Using a very broad definition, the prevalence of live births affected by atypical sex characteristics has been estimated to be as high as 1 in 200 (Blackless et al. 2000).

Diverse sex development is not limited to babies presenting genital ambiguity that renders gender assignment difficult. It is, for example, relatively common for men and boys to be born with the urethral opening at the base or on the shaft of the penis rather than at the tip. More rarely, some men have a single testis, and some have testes that are "vanishing." Some men present for fertility investigations only to be told that they have uterine and ovarian structures and are potentially capable of menstruation. Some girls do not menstruate in their teens. Clinical investigations may identify in some girls "ovarian insufficiency," in other girls healthy ovaries but no womb, cervix, or vagina, and, in still others, abdominal testes and a male-typical chromosomal karyotype. For reasons not well understood, some boys and girls do not go into puberty spontaneously, and some present signs of puberty in early childhood. There is actually no need to look to people with identified genetic variations for atypical sex characteristics. In the general population, for example, many healthy men have breasts and many healthy women do not; furthermore many healthy men have very little facial or body hair and many healthy women have a lot.

Advances in biotechnology have contributed to the identification of an increasing number of genetic links to atypical sex characteristics. A few years ago, an international group of experts revised and standardized the nomenclature, to make future biomedical research more expedient. The result was the first and only international consensus statement.

An umbrella term, "disorders of sex development," was put forward as a way to denote a broad range of diagnoses; that is, to include all "congenital conditions in which development of chromosomal, gonadal or anatomical sex is atypical" (Hughes, Houk, Lee, Ahmed, & LWPES/ESPE Consensus Group 2006).

In parallel with increasing interests in molecular biology, the range of conditions covered by the term is widening to include sex-chromosome aneuploidies that may not be associated with anomalies of the external genitalia or gonadal failure (e.g., XXY or XO mosaicism).

All terms used to describe body differences are potentially pejorative, and all of them can be expected to cause offence. It is unsurprising that "disorders of sex development" has been greeted with mixed reactions (Hughes et al. 2006 [Responses]; Davis, 2011). For the purpose of this chapter, we refer to these same conditions as *diverse sex development* (DSD), to acknowledge the fact that many affected individuals consider their bodies different rather than disordered.

"Sex" is often equated with the biological and is expressed in dimorphic terms, whereas "gender" has been introduced to denote the psychosocial and behavioral. Biological factors are generally believed to contribute to gender identity, but the importance of biology is positioned very differently across disciplines. "Gender" is a concept that is meant to transcend binary categorization. But, just like "sex," it, too, is expressed in dimorphic terms. "Sex" and "gender" are thus often used interchangeably. Our restrictive language is unable to do justice to human diversity in body, identity, and behavior. Experts in gender studies say that it is no accident that we have been strongly taught to assume that body, identity, and sexuality are binary and mutually exclusive when they are best thought of as continuous. These distortions contribute to clinical communication challenges in the DSD field. The majority of people, regardless of age, race, class, religion, disability, and sexuality, take for granted that there are two types of bodies—male and female. The fact that most bodies tend to be more or less male-typical or more or less female-typical is given little thought. It is therefore not surprising that bodies with both male-typical and female-typical features are greeted with surprise.

In recent years, medical management of these bodies has been the subject of intense debates, triggered not least by dissatisfied and aggrieved adult service users. The debates raise profound issues about the purpose of maintaining sex and gender dichotomies in the face of bodies and identities that challenge them; about the ethics of normalizing genital surgery on infants and children with body differences; about medical and parental power; about informed consent; and about how best to assist people caught between the benefits and costs of normative embodiment and resistance to it (Liao and Boyle, 2004). Given such uncertainties, the importance of optimal clinical communication should be obvious.

In this chapter, suggestions for improved clinical communications are offered, with the tacit acknowledgment that these interventions would have limited values without a collective effort to interrogate (hetero)normative embodiment. Our suggestions are informed by the work that we have done with and for people with a range of DSD diagnoses, with clinical examples drawn mainly though not exclusively on women with XY conditions. We believe that our recommendations for sensitive exploration that is founded on continued scrutiny of our own inevitably value-laden perceptions are relevant to a much broader range of clinical situations that challenge people's sense of maleness and femaleness (e.g., consulting to women post-mastectomy). Molecular research of atypical sex characteristics may separate people into categories, but the communication challenges for care providers in different specialties and for differently labeled service users have much in common.

BACKGROUND

Diagnosis of genetic conditions associated with DSD may be made at any age, sometimes along with other body differences or health problems. When the external genitalia appear ambiguous (e.g., the clitoris is sufficiently enlarged to appear like a small penis, or the labia are sufficiently fused to give a scrotal appearance), diagnosis of the underlying condition is often made in infancy. When the external genitalia look typical but the internal genitalia do not (e.g., absent or small vagina and/or uterus, presence of intra-abdominal testes in a girl), the underlying condition may not be identified until adolescence (e.g., following investigations for primary amenorrhea). In the case of childhood presentation, most individuals would have come under medical management. The pediatric specialists most likely to assume clinical responsibilities are endocrinologists and urologists.

When genital differences are detected, virtually all children with a known female karyotype are assigned female, and feminizing genital surgery usually ensues; children with a known male karyotype whose penis is absent or very small are also likely to be assigned female (Creighton & Liao 2004).

DSD conditions are too numerous to mention. Therefore, only two of the better known conditions are briefly described here. Androgen insensitivity syndrome (AIS) affects only fetuses with male-typical karyotype (XY). The fetus produces typical amounts of androgens but lacks receptors to respond to them. In its "complete" form (CAIS), the infant typically presents female external genitalia, hence the condition may not be diagnosed until adolescence, usually prompted by absence of menstruation. In its partial form (PAIS), the individual is born with genitalia that are virilized to a greater or less extent. People with AIS do not have ovaries, womb, or cervix, and instead have testicular gonads and a vagina that is shorter than average. Until relatively recently, concealment of the diagnosis from CAIS and other XY females was typical, in the interest of psychological adjustment. Case Study 1 represents this type of scenario in a client with an XY female condition known as pure XY gonadal dysgenesis or Swyer syndrome. Health professionals in genetics may be required not only to help newly diagnosed clients assimilate complex medical information and process its impact on their sense of self, they may also need to take special care to eliminate further communication mishaps in older clients working through the emotional burden of having been deceived (see Box 3.1).

A second, better known DSD diagnosis is congenital adrenal hyperplasia (CAH), a metabolic condition that affects XX and XY babies. In this situation, the fetus is exposed to unusually high levels of prenatal androgens. An XX infant would have a womb, upper vagina, ovaries, and fertility potential and also present partially virilized external genitalia. Fertility potential has primacy in gender assignment. Therefore, most XX babies with CAH are assigned female.

In most cases of ambiguous genitalia, surgery is carried out to "feminize" the genitals, even for children who are known to be genetically male but whose penis is believed to be too small for them to be successfully reared as males. The greater emphasis on female sex assignment has partly been influenced by the lesser technical

Box 3.1 Case Study 1

In 2011, a 50-year-old woman contacted the Androgen Insensitivity Syndrome Support Group (AISSG) UK in some distress. She had been seen by her family doctor at age 14, when periods had not started, and, at age 17, laparoscopic investigations identified "streak ovaries" (streaks of undeveloped and inactive gonadal tissue typical for Swyer syndrome) and she was told that she could never have children. When training as a nurse, she had bloods taken and was told that she had "an extra male chromosome." The implications were not explained to her (she subsequently found "XY karyotype not disclosed" written in her medical notes). At 21 she had a "gonadectomy," with the same family doctor citing a cancer risk as the reason. She then attended an endocrine clinic once a year and started on hormone replacement therapy (HRT).

The identification of defects of the aorta and near blood vessels in 2010 led her to consult a gynecologist to discuss stopping HRT. This clinician confirmed the diagnosis of Swyer syndrome, which means she has a uterus and might have been able to sustain a pregnancy via in vitro fertilization and egg donation. She has missed out on potential fertility treatment and genetic counseling.

In her extended dialogue with AISSG, she said, "I had pieces of the jigsaw but the lack of a name did mean that I couldn't put it all together." She referred to "the existential crisis I have been in, as to who I now am, with this new info."

difficulty of constructing genitals that can be penetrated than genitals that can penetrate (Chase, 1998a). Such surgery is usually carried out in the first 2 months of life and no later than 2 years, with the intention of providing secure gender identity and psychological adjustment and of relieving parents of what is assumed to be an intolerable burden of uncertainty (Liao & Boyle 2004). Following gender assignment and surgical sexing of the genitals, it has been traditional practice to recommend secrecy or at least incomplete disclosure to the child or siblings, again in the interest of psychological adjustment.

"Feminizing" surgery is without exception invasive and may include any or all of the following: reduction of the external clitoris (the visible part), refashioning of the labia, or reconstruction of the vagina. Children cannot consent to the elective surgery. Furthermore, research with adults suggests that surgery often has to be repeated, and that, contrary to pediatric claims, appearance and functional and sexual outcomes are unsatisfactory in adults (Creighton, Minto, & Steele 2001; Crouch et al. 2008; Minto, Liao, Conway, & Creighton, 2003). Normalizing genital surgery is avoided in male-assigned babies, because doctors are much less confident about phalloplasties on babies and young children, and tissues are preserved for procedures in adolescence and adulthood.

It may come as a surprise that the availability of (the small number of) designated adult DSD services is a relatively recent provision in the United Kingdom. Until a decade or so ago, clients discharged from pediatric services were lost to follow-up, and little was known about how they fared in the adult world. Any effort to examine the effects of the interventionist surgical care protocol has tended to focus on whether the individual changes gender later on. The implicit assumption was that if people did not reassign gender in adulthood, then the interventions were justified. So confident were doctors about childhood normalizing genital surgery that its social, emotional, and sexual benefits and harms were left unexamined for several decades.

Criticisms levied at the medical profession in recent years have focused on the withholding of diagnostic information, nonconsensual surgery, the absence of follow-up evaluations, and inadequate psychological support (e.g. Anonymous 1994; Chase 1998b; Simmonds 2004). It is now recognized that the best care is multidisciplinary and one that incorporates consumer views. Improved access to psychological care for people with so-called disorders of sex development has been proposed since the mid-1990s. However, service delivery—its theoretical frameworks, service priorities, and methods—have never been coherently articulated (Liao 2007; Liao & Simmonds, in press).

PREPARING FOR THE CONSULTATION

Because of the stigma attached to DSD, service users can be expected to be highly variable in their relationship to the diagnosis. Some service users would find it aversive to ask for directions to "the DSD Clinic." The name of the clinic reflects the user-centeredness of the service. Choice exists in naming the clinic for example after a user advocate or the name of the local area.

DSD diagnoses are numerous but each is rare. Therefore, it is unrealistic to expect clinic staff to be familiar with the details of DSD conditions. Training for ancillary staff, such as receptionists, radiographers, and outpatient nurses, should focus on basic etiquette, such as not openly discussing the purpose of the appointment and calling out or displaying the client's clinic number rather than his or her full name. Some service users may choose to use a pseudonym. This choice is often made in the interest of partners and/or family members who prefer to remain anonymous. Having to share a waiting area with pregnant women, or where walls are plastered with baby photographs, can be painful for some DSD clients, as can being asked about their last period or cervical smear test by an intake nurse in front of other people.

Box 3.2 contains an excerpt from an article that appeared in the *British Medical Journal* by an anonymous woman with CAIS who has this to say about how poor communications added to her "despair."

> **Box 3.2**
>
> I was admitted to hospital for adhesions and a nurse asked me if I had previously had a penis. I was seen by a psychiatrist in his office in a maternity hospital with a heavily pregnant doctor participating. I was seen by a psychosexual counsellor who tried to take me apart and reconstruct my psyche, a process which nearly caused a mental breakdown. (Anonymous 1994)

The team needs to decide on who the best person is to welcome the client or family at their first visit. This person may be a nurse, a psychologist, or a service coordinator. A few minutes spent in preparing the client or family for the consultation can help the client or family to reach a state of relative calm by the time they meet the medical consultant. Inquiry about the journey, about hopes and concerns regarding the appointment, about the most important questions at the forefront of their minds, can help the client or family to feel that they are attending a service that is sufficiently developed to anticipate their preoccupations. The first contact person can also offer the client or family information about the clinic and individual team members, and the order of events and their scheduling. Photographs of team members in the waiting room can help to "humanize" the service immediately.

DSD is seldom discussed in everyday life, so the tertiary center that clients attend may be the only safe place where all aspects of their conditions can be freely and openly discussed. Care providers should not underestimate the high value placed by service users on a robust professional alliance.

COMMUNICATING IN THE CONSULTATION: TALKING TO PARENTS ABOUT THEIR CHILD'S DSD

Adults with DSD conditions suggest that parents need to "come to terms" with the diagnoses themselves in order to help their children (Simmonds 2004). When presented with a child with non-normative sex development, however, parents can be expected to feel extremely confused and emotionally vulnerable. "Coming to terms" may require sustained support for coping with losses and fears, and for examining our taken-for-granted beliefs about "normal sexuality" and "normal life."

Health professionals' behaviors can be expected to be highly influential on their client's sense-making of the situation. Every clinician meeting the parents for the first time should begin with congratulating the parents on the arrival of their baby and then engage them in the usual exchanges about their baby and about being parents (again). When there is a delay in gender assignment, it is important to listen to the parents' reactions without rushing to placate them (see Box 3.3).

It can be reassuring for parents to know that, although they had not come across these situations, the situations are not so uncommon. The message that DSD is at least as common as twins or red hair may be easier to relate to than prevalence in numerical terms. The professional and reliable presence of an understanding and expert team will help to contain emotions.

There may be further investigations to implement. If not urgent, then the client or family should be allowed sufficient time to absorb the information in order to make an informed choice. Medical preoccupations may not be in synch with what is occupying the client's mind. Here are some example questions to elicit information on how the parents are processing the event:

- These are some very clinical words, what do they mean to you? What effects do these words have on you?
- Who is able to support you; are there others whose support you need?
- How do you see this affecting how you feel about yourself? And your child?
- In what way will your relationships change, in what way will they remain the same?
- How would you like other people to understand this condition? What words would you use? Can we help?
- How would you describe the way you're feeling right now? What can we do to help?

Box 3.3

A set of guidelines (DSD Guidelines 2006) provides an example wording, which we have modified here:

"Your baby was born with a kind of variation that happens more often than you hear about. Our team works with these situations regularly. We are doing a series of tests to find out whether your baby is probably going to feel more like a boy or a girl. We expect to have more information for you within [realistic timeframe]. Although you may not feel ready to send out a birth announcement with the baby's gender and name, there are some choices to consider, such as letting close friends and families know that you have a healthy baby who is full of personality, or send photographs to show how lovely your baby is, or let them know how best to support you."

Gender Assignment in Infancy

Aside from the diagnostic information and prognostic projections, parental preference for gender assignment may be informed by familial, cultural, and religious values, and whether there are already boys and girls within the family. Other parents want to know the "true sex" of their child and whether their child will grow up to be a happy individual. Parents may be reassured that the same conditions that enable children to thrive are exactly the same as those that enable children with DSD to thrive.

Parents may ask if their child would be "normal" in relationships. This type of question offers opportunities for the team to help the parents to "unpack" what "normal" means, and what they value most about relationships. Implicit in questions about normal relationships is whether their child will be homosexual. Some parents may feel unsure about asking this question, perhaps because they are afraid to hear what they think might be the answer, or perhaps because they worry about offending the clinician to whom they are talking. It is important to anticipate the concern and assist the clients to find the words, so that the issues can be openly discussed. It is not possible to predict any child's future sexuality, and the majority of gay people do not have a DSD condition. Whichever direction their sexuality takes, young people will benefit from the same support and acceptance.

Perhaps the most important message to offer parents is that they are not alone, that other families have worked with the same situation. Today, parents can potentially access Internet support from all over the world, or telephone or face-to-face contact with peer groups (e.g., AISSG; DSDfamilies).

Feminizing Genital Surgery for Female-Assigned Children

Feminizing surgery does not improve the child's health, therefore it is a difficult choice for parents to make on behalf of their daughter. Good intentions of care providers are not a replacement for thorough exploration that gives equal weight to immediate surgery and delaying surgery until the child can participate in the decision process. Care providers must avoid subtly pressuring parents to make a decision before they have had enough time to bond with their child and to digest all of the information or consult with support groups if they wish. Clinicians should be prepared to discuss the pros and cons of potential interventions, answer any questions, and even refer for a second opinion if the parents are finding it too difficult to reach a balanced decision that they are comfortable with.

Whatever parents choose, they do so in the interest of the child. Those who choose surgery may be motivated by the expectation that surgery will normalize their daughter's genital appearance and that she will be spared any ridicule or rejection. They may believe that it will encourage a female gender identify. They may also believe that their concerns about sharing information with babysitters, helpers, and teachers about the child's diagnosis will be removed. It is important to be clear about how realistic these expectations are. Normalizing surgery does not eliminate the diagnosis. Their psychological engagement with the issues will continue to be required.

Discussion of the short-term risks and long-term uncertainties will help parents make what is a stressful and perhaps traumatic decision that they will have to live with. Pediatric surgeons are generally more optimistic about surgery than are adult care providers. One reason for the schism is that the former will follow-up infants and children for short periods—before puberty and engagement in sexual relationships—whereas the latter see postpubertal adolescents and adults who have been operated on as children, often repeatedly and with poor outcomes. It is recommended that pediatric doctors inform parents that surgery is highly unlikely to be one-off, and that there is a debate about satisfactory outcomes in terms of appearance and function in adulthood.

For the currently small proportion of parents who decide to defer surgery until their child can give consent, psychological input for communication skills development is needed. The parents may need to educate not just the affected child but also siblings and the extended family or wider community; in other words, they will need help in developing a more constructive, systemic approach for education about non-normative sex development in the child.

Intimate Examinations and Photography

Children who are operated on are especially vulnerable to repeated genital examinations and photography because doctors are compelled to monitor and evidence results. Some pediatricians have alluded to the "repeated psychological insult caused by frequent genital examinations and operations" (Jaaslekainen, Tiitimen, & Voutilainen 2001), and some gynecologists and psychologists have warned about the emotional distress caused by medical photography (Creighton, Alderson, Brown, & Minto 2002). Genital surgery for ambiguous genitalia is intended to normalize gender identity and sexuality but, ironically, the attendant scrutiny that follows surgery is a direct challenge to the psychological justification for it.

Small developmentally appropriate steps can be taken to reduce the shame and embarrassment associated with intimate examinations and photography:

- The presence of any observer must be rationalized with a tacit assumption that families will feel under a great deal of pressure to comply with doctors whose good will is important to them. The family should always have the benefit of the slightest doubt.

- Invite the child to bring his or her favorite toy or object of comfort.
- Give time for the family to settle.
- Involve the child rather than distract him or her to avoid possible dissociation under stress that could lead to future psychological problems.
- Invite child and parents to ask any questions concerning the necessity and nature of the examinations and photography.
- Offer choices to provide a sense of control (e.g., invite the child to choose a gown, whether he or she would prefer the doctor to stand to the right or left, and so on).
- Start with other parts of the body (e.g., feet, fingers, ears). Invite the child to do the same for his or her doll or teddy bear likewise, to find out how doll or teddy is doing.
- Invite the child to use the stethoscope to check if the doctor is well.
- In case of photography, provide a toy camera for the child to take pictures of the adults present.
- In nonurgent situations, offer a genuine choice as to whether the child or family would prefer to have the examination or photography at the next appointment.

The existence of a protocol for intimate examination and photography and the care that goes into it reflects the team's collective awareness of psychological risks and respect for emotional safety for the child. Every photography occasion should have a rational basis—what is it for, what should be the timing, how should the client or family be prepared to maximize perceived control, dignity, and respect?

Counseling Parents About Risks of the Same Diagnosis in Future Pregnancies

DSD conditions differ in the extent to which a known genetic component is implicated. In an X-linked recessive condition such as AIS, there is a 1 in 4 chance in a given pregnancy of an XY boy, an XY AIS child, an XX girl or an XX carrier girl. A range of mutations on the androgen receptor (AR) gene has been identified, and most, if not all, cases of CAIS can be explained by receptor defects. However, the majority of PAIS individuals exhibit no defect in androgen-receptor binding, suggesting that other genetic defects are involved. It is also possible in PAIS for the same genetic defect to express itself as differing genital appearances. CAIS and PAIS may thus be caused by different defects at the genetic/cellular level and are thought not to occur in the same family (Ahmed et al. 2000). Also, in about a half to one-third of cases, AIS arises from a de novo mutation. In some of the other XY female DSDs, such as Swyer syndrome, 5-alpha-reductase deficiency, and Leydig cell hypoplasia, a role of genetic in the condition has not been established with any certainty.

At a time when the AR gene and its mutations were being actively researched (up to the late 1990s), families in the United Kingdom would have to persuade a research team to carry out carrier testing as a favor on the back of their research, there being no National Health Service (NHS) testing service available. This was a long and frustrating process for some families, as illustrated in Box 3.4, which was provided by a family who welcomed genetic testing but were unable to access the service.

The Androgen Insensitivity Syndrome Support Group (AISSG) UK has received inquiries from parents of newborn babies with AIS who are angry that they have only now discovered that older female relatives had kept to themselves facts about their own AIS (with or without knowledge of its inherited nature) for many years. Conversely, there have been enquiries from older adult women who have been prompted, by the birth of an AIS baby into the wider family (in an era when parents are more likely to have received truthful disclosure and to be more active in seeking out information), to look into the reason for their own failure to menstruate and consequent infertility. There have also been cases in which a woman seeking AIS carrier testing, at the time when this was done in a research laboratory, was surprised and somewhat alarmed to discover that the researchers had been aware of AIS in her

---

Box 3.4 Case Study 2

In 2012, Androgen Insensitivity Syndrome Support Group (AISSG) UK was contacted by a 36 year-old woman with complete androgen insensitivity syndrome (CAIS). She was diagnosed at 12 months of age, following a left inguinal hernia, but did not find out about her diagnosis until she was 27 years old.

She has an older brother and two older XX female sisters. Her genetic testing to confirm CAIS had helped her sisters to get tested for carrier status. She explained, "My middle sister, who already had a girl [now aged 12] and two boys, is not a carrier. However my oldest sister is a carrier…I think her IVF was out of necessity (she was 40) and not due to her being a carrier for AIS. Her daughter [aged 18 months] was conceived from a donor egg so there is no chance of her being affected by AIS."

In relation to genetic risks, this woman said: "because I didn't know [about the diagnosis], neither did my sisters…who could then have been carriers, so then my [middle] sister's daughter could have had it too. And again, when my sister wanted to find out in advance [if she might be a carrier], the consultant she saw was very anti finding out and told her that her daughter had a right not to know and that even if she turned out to be a carrier he would not test her daughter."

When asked if her story could be used in this chapter, she said: "I would be extremely happy for you to use my story in any way which you think it might bring an end to all this nonsense of doctors/parents keeping critical medical information from clients and their families."

family members for many years, even though she was the first to have sought such testing.

In a different scenario, invitation to genetic testing could fill the client with dread of having to disclose and discuss DSD within the family. A collaborative approach that safeguards informed consent means plenty of time and opportunities to help clients explore the potential implications of genetic testing for family relationships, as well as education and support for potential carriers to appreciate the implications (including the communication challenges with the next generation).

Advice to Parents About Talking to the Growing Child

Far from protecting the child, narratives by affected adults and psychological research suggest that lying, evasive answers, and refusal to discuss DSD is potentially psychologically harmful to the affected growing child.

It is imperative that parents are open and honest about their child's DSD, and clinicians should take it upon themselves to lead by example and communicate in no uncertain terms that DSD is nothing to be ashamed of. However, although openness and honesty signals to the child that he or she is fully accepted without shame, parents differ in how resourced they are for meeting the communication challenges. A central concern for parents is what message to give to the child about what he or she should do with the information. Thus, disclosure about DSD may feel like a floodgate that has to be either fully closed or fully opened.

In tolerating and accepting clients' distress, even if it feels overwhelming at times, clinicians are nurturing the clients' capacity for the emotionally charged and risky task of talking to their child and other family members about DSD. In sharing information about DSD, parents are more likely to be able to access social support and end their isolation. Conversely, if parents are poorly cared for by the clinical team, their capacity for open communication may be diminished and, in time, their fear and shame may be magnified.

COMMUNICATING WITH THE ADOLESCENT AND ADULT CLIENT

The following excerpt, from the *British Medical Journal* article mentioned earlier, illustrates very well our rigid dimorphic view of gender that is so unhelpful to people with DSD. There are no easy solutions to this problem, but a supported exploration of the identity issues provides a space where clients can begin to develop their own responses.

I am chromosomally male, a pseudo-hermaphrodite. These two phrases pervaded my rational thought. I did not think I was female. I did not think I was male. I did not know what I was. (Anonymous 1994)

Diagnosis

As mentioned earlier, some DSD diagnoses are reached during adolescence, a time when people tend to be highly sensitive about social norms in bodies and their appearances. Affected adolescents and adults are likely to be devastated when told of their diagnosis. Their self-evaluations may be compromised by dominant stories of "normality" and "abnormality" about sex and sexuality in the social world, stories that position their situation as "deviant."

Any of the following diagnostic information, delivered in a clinical language, can be shocking: absent vagina, absent menstruation, infertility, chromosomes, heredity, lifelong medication, hirsutism, weight gain, and short stature. An important first task then, is to develop a shared language with clients. Questions such as the following may be helpful for starting a discussion:

- What words would you prefer to use?
- What's the most challenging aspect of your situation to put into words?

Clinicians can be overly focused on medical information, when it is the meaning that determines reactions. Communication of the diagnostic and treatment information in plain language needs to be followed by empathic engagement with the young person's emotional reactions, which needs to be followed by the development of richer vocabularies drawn on alternative discourses to address the social, emotional, and sexual aspects of DSD.

Questions such as the following may be helpful for exploring the client's understanding of the condition and, should they be necessary, treatment options:

- Can you tell me the name of the diagnosis? What kind of information have you been given about this?
- What have you been told about the investigations that are happening and what they are for?
- What is your understanding of how the tests fit with your overall treatment plan?
- How would you describe the way you're feeling right now?

The following questions may be helpful for extending the dialogue:

- What effects do these long words have on you?
- How would you like other people to understand this?
- If you were to brainstorm different words, what might you come up with?

Decision About Genital (Re)constructive Surgery

Where a gender boundary is blurred by characteristics deemed to belong to the "opposite sex", individuals can become extremely preoccupied with fixing the problem.

Many women with DSD diagnoses speak of feeling like outsiders and feeling unentitled to relationships until they have had surgery, such as vaginoplasty, to remove the obstacles for "normal sex" (Boyle et al. 2005). When clients seek medical treatment, they may also be seeking "normality" in identity, relationships, and sexual practices. Health professionals feel under a great deal of pressure to ensure that diagnostic information simultaneously comes with offers of some form of a normality solution. But, although this may help to contain doctor and client anxiety, such action inadvertently comes with the subtext that body differences are unacceptable, indeed inconceivable—even for a minute. It is this subtext that is ultimately unhelpful.

Decision to undergo surgery may be fear-based—to avoid the need to explain about DSD. It is possible to further the client's understanding of the benefits and limitations of any treatment, for example, by asking:

- Can you repeat to me in your own words what you have been told about the treatment—what is the procedure called, what does it involve, how long does the operation take, what is the recovery period?
- What do you understand to be the potential benefits and risks—immediately and in the longer term?
- Which aspects of your life are dependent on the operation? Which aspects are more up to you?
- Who else can help you reach a balanced decision not just about treatment but the best timing for you?
- What do you think the operation may leave unaddressed? What else might be needed? What steps would you take? Who else can help?

Fertility Issues

In many cases of XY female DSD conditions, there is a fundamental infertility because of interrupted gonadal development and lack of a uterus; however in those with Swyer syndrome, the presence of a primitive uterus can sometimes, with hormone treatment, lead to menstruation and pregnancy using in vitro fertilization (IVF) and a donor egg. The case study in Box 3.5 illustrates an acute need for better communication about genetics.

Genetic Research

In the current race toward molecular discoveries, scientists and clinicians may not have developed sufficient appreciation of the potentially far-reaching implications that genetic testing can have for some clients and their relationships with self and others. We have met clients who felt torn by having to discuss their DSD, which was a family taboo, but for whom such discussion was necessary to involve generations of family members in genetic research as a token of gratitude to their doctors. Genetic

Box 3.5 Case Study 3

A "female with partial androgen insensitivity syndrome (PAIS)" who has two affected sisters, all of whom were said to have inherited the condition from their father, recently contacted Androgen Insensitivity Syndrome Support Group (AISSG) UK One of the sisters had two children, including a son with PAIS. The inquirer had been trying unsuccessfully to have children for 3 years. Both she and husband had been fully tested and received the "all-clear." She said, "I never mentioned the genetic condition to my doctors as I didn't think it made a difference at this point. However, I am now wondering if this could affect my chances of conception?"

When it was pointed out that AIS is usually passed on via the mother (if inherited, as opposed to being a de novo mutation) and that women with PAIS do not have ovaries or uterus, and do not menstruate, so cannot conceive, the inquirer replied:

"My dad has the PAIS. As it is his X that is affected, he passed on his bad X (so to speak) to me and my two sisters. Us three sisters have all been told by a genetic counsellor that we all have 50% good X and 50% bad X and have all had a blood test to confirm this. My nephew, now aged 8, inherited the bad X off my sister, who has also been confirmed and diagnosed as having PAIS; my nephew has had countless operations to try and correct the hypospadias on his penis. My sister with PAIS has had children and I have had scans and have all internal and external female organs. We have been told that as carriers of PAIS, females are only affected by having less pubic hair. It only came to light that me and my two sisters had this when my nephew was born and tested. We have definitely got PAIS and all have a 1 in 2 chance of passing this on to our children."

An XY male fathered by a man with androgen insensitivity could not have inherited his father's X chromosome, and thus would neither inherit nor carry the gene for the syndrome. A genetic female conceived in such a way would have inherited her father's X chromosome, and would thus become a carrier. A female carrier has a 50% chance of passing the affected androgen receptor (AR) gene to her children. If the affected child is a genetic female, she too will be a carrier; and an affected 46,XY child will have AIS. Therefore, it was explained to this woman that she and her sisters must have been XX females who are *carriers* of the faulty gene inherited from their PAIS father; that they did not *have* PAIS, because only people with an XY karyotype could have PAIS. They could not be both a carrier of, and be affected by, AIS—it had to be one or the other. It was recommended that they seek advice about any possible effect on the fertility of carriers.

The case study illustrates the complexity of genetic to lay people, and the importance of developing creative and multimedia means of communication, rather than relying solely on verbal exchanges and literacy. Level of understanding needs to be carefully explored in genetic counseling, which offers opportunities for previous misconceptions to be corrected and for clients to be signposted to seek appropriate advice on important issues such as fertility.

testing can be a driver for first-time disclosure within the extended family. Although this can be a positive process, the client needs to be ready and must be doing this for him- or herself. Where there is a sibling with the same diagnosis, one individual's decision will profoundly affect the other, who may view the process in hostile terms. We have come across significant conflict between affected siblings because of genetic testing. Professional psychological support is typically not considered necessary.

Because people affected by DSD have historically been poorly served by their care providers, genetic researchers whose work is less than likely to benefit the affected individual must work within the strictest ethical and professional governance frameworks.

SUMMARY

Bodies that challenge our erroneous binary categorizations of sex and gender have always existed. They have come under professional and scientific scrutiny for only a short period of time, relative to the thousands of years of their recorded history. The socially sanctioned project of bioclassification and normalization of atypically sexed bodies is replete with controversies and schisms. At one end of the polarity, bio banks are being built to study molecular causes of "abnormal" reproductive and genital development, mainly to improve understanding of "normal" development. At the other end, the very notion of "normality" is understood as a social construct that suits specific temporal and cultural locations. Somewhere within this spectrum of knowledge production sits medical management of atypically sexed bodies.

Space does not permit a full exposition of research and practice ethics in the field. Nevertheless, we hope we have provided sufficient context to argue for a swing toward a client-centered approach to clinical management and research and have signposted to the critical importance of robust communication skills in such a service model. Elsewhere, we argue that there is sufficient negative user feedback to warrant the development of in-depth communication training for clinicians in the field (Liao & Simmonds, in press). Meanwhile, here is a summary list of points that we think clinicians should bear in mind in terms of communicating about DSD:

- Always privilege emotional safety, dignity, and respect for the client.
- Be aware of one's own personal values and assumptions relating to "normality" in sex and sexuality and their influence on professional practice.
- Role model shame-free communication about DSD that enables rather than diminishes the client.
- Speak in relative rather than absolute terms (e.g., "variations" and "difference" instead of "normal" and "abnormal," "shorter than average" instead of "short," "unwanted hair growth" instead of "hirsutism").

- Tailor communication to the age, developmental stage, and current emotional well-being of the client.
- Check understanding, expectations, and feelings relating to aspects of the diagnosis and any procedures.
- Encourage balanced decision making in relation to elective procedures.
- Provide information about user support organizations.

Routine collection of anonymous client feedback is a tangible way to involve clients in ongoing service improvement. It offers them opportunities to express their appreciation of the team and the organization.

REFERENCES

Ahmed, S. F., Cheng, A., Dovey, L., Hawkins, J. R., Martin, J., Rowland, J., et al. (2000). Phenotypic features, androgen receptor binding and mutational analysis in 278 clinical cases reported as androgen insensitivity syndrome. *Journal of Clinical Endocrinology and Metabolism, 85*(2), 658–665.

Androgen Insensitivity Syndrome Support Group (AISSG): http://www.aissg.org

Anonymous. (1994, February). Once a dark secret. *British Medical Journal*. Response letters in April, 1994 issue.

Blackless, M. Charuvastra, A., Derryck, A., Fausto-Sterling, A., Lauzanne, K., et al. (2000). How sexually dimorphic are we? Review and synthesis. *American Journal of Human Biology, 12,*151–166.

Boyle, M., Smith, S., & Liao, L.-M. (2005). Adult genital surgery for intersex women: a solution to what problem? *Journal of Health Psychology, 10,* 573–584.

Chase, C. (1998a). Surgical progress not the answer to intersexuality. *Journal of Clinical Ethics, 9*(4): 385–392.

Chase, C. (1998b). Affronting reason. In D. Atkins (Ed.), *Looking queer: Image and identity in lesbian, bisexual, gay and transgendered communities* (pp. 205–219). Binghamton, NY: Haworth.

Creighton, S. M., Alderson, J., Brown, S., & Minto, C. L. (2002). Medical photography: Ethics, consent and the intersex patient. *British Journal of Urology International, 89,* 67–72.

Creighton, S. M., & Liao, L.-M. (2004). Changing attitudes to sex assignment in intersex. *British Journal of Urology International, 93*(5), 659–664.

Creighton, S. M., Minto, C. L., & Steele, S. J. (2001). Objective cosmetic and anatomical outcomes at adolescence of feminising surgery for ambiguous genitalia done in childhood. *The Lancet, 358* (July 14), 124–125.

Crouch, N. S., Liao, L.-M. Woodhouse, C. R. J., Conway, G. S., & Creighton, S. M. (2008). Genital sensitivity and sexual function following childhood cosmetic genital surgery: Results based on women with congenital adrenal hyperplasia. *Journal of Urology, 179*(2), 634–638.

Davis, G. (2011). 'DSD is a perfectly fine term': Reasserting medical authority through a shift in intersex terminology. In P. J. McGann & D. J. Hutson (Eds.), *Sociology of diagnosis, issue of advances in medical sociology* (Vol. 12, pp.155–182). Bingley, UK: Emerald Group Publishing Limited.

Dreger, A. D., Chase, C., Sousa, A., Gruppuso, P. A., & Frader, J. (2005). Changing the nomenclature/taxonomy for intersex: A scientific and clinical rationale. *Journal of Pediatric Endocrinology and Metabolism, 18*, 729–733.

DSDfamilies (resource for parents and teenagers). Available at http://www.dsdfamilies.org

DSD Guidelines. (2006). Published by DSD Consortium. Available at http://www.accordalliance.org/dsd-guidelines.html

Hughes, I. A. (2002). Intersex. *British Journal of Urology International, 90*, 769–776.

Hughes, I. A., Houk, C., Ahmed, S. F., Lee, P. A., & LWPES/ESPE Consensus Group. (2006). Consensus statement on management of intersex disorders. *Archives of Disease in Childhood, 91*, 554–563. Article and responses available at http://adc.bmj.com/content/91/7/554

Jaaslekainen, J., Tiitimen, A., & Voutilainen, R. (2001). Sexual function and fertility in adult females and males with congenital adrenal hyperplasia. *Hormone Research, 56*, 73–80.

Liao, L. -M. (2007). Towards a clinical-psychological approach to address the hetero sexual concerns of intersexed women. In V. Clarke & E. Peel (Eds.), *Out in psychology: Lesbian, gay, bisexual and transgender perspectives* (pp. 391–408). New York: Wiley.

Liao, L.-M., & Boyle, M. (2004). Intersex. *The Psychologist, 17*(8), 446–447.

Liao, L.-M., & Simmonds, M. (in press). A values-driven and evidence-based health care psychology for diverse sex development. *Psychology & Sexuality.*

Minto, C. L., Liao, L.-M., Conway, G. S., & Creighton, S. M. (2003). Sexual function in women with complete androgen insensitivity syndrome. *Fertility and Sterility, 8*(1), 157–164.

Simmonds, M. (2004). Patients and parents in decision making and management. In A. H. Balen, S. M. Creighton, M. C. Davies, J. MacDougall, & R. Stanhope (Eds.), *Paediatric and adolescent gynaecology—A multidisciplinary approach* (pp. 205–228). Cambridge University Press.

4 Communicating with Clients from the Jewish Community

Sara Levene

"A wise man hears one word and understands two."
—*Yiddish proverb*

This chapter aims to place Jewish clients in the context of their community and wider, and to address some of the Jewish cultural and religious issues that may be relevant at the interface with clinical genetics. However, many of the issues covered are most relevant when counseling Orthodox and ultra-Orthodox families, for whom cultural and religious traditions will have the most impact on decision making.

BACKGROUND

Ethnic Jewish Groups

In terms of ethnic differences that affect susceptibilities to common founder mutations, the main groups are Ashkenazi and Sephardi Jews. Until the year 70 of the Common Era (known in the Christian world as 70 AD), the Jewish world was largely resident in the ancient land of Israel. Central to Jewish life in the ancient land of Israel was the Temple in Jerusalem. However, it was around this time that the Romans destroyed the Temple, and, following this event, the Jewish population started to disperse.

After several centuries, the Jews gradually migrated northward into the German region of Ashkenaz and later migrated across Northern and Eastern Europe. This

Note on pronunciations of Yiddish and Hebrew words: "ch" is always pronounced as in a Scottish "loch."

group has become known as Ashkenazi (Ash-ken-ah-zi). With the rise of Nazism in the 20th century, large numbers of this population fled Europe to North America, Britain, modern-day Israel, and other parts of the world.

The Sephardi (Sef-ar-di) population originates from those groups that settled in Spain and Portugal after the destruction of the Temple. During the Spanish Inquisition of 1492, many of the Jewish population were expelled from these lands and migrated to North Africa, Turkey, and Arabic-speaking countries, as well as to other parts of Europe. Parts of North Africa and the Arab world also had their own indigenous Jewish populations (Mizrahi [Miz-ra-hi] Jews), with which the Sephardim assimilated. In modern times, it is common to refer to all Jews from North African or Arabic-speaking countries as Sephardim, and, on the whole, they practice common customs. However, in Israel, the term "Mizrahi" is also used distinctly to describe Eastern and Oriental Jews who do not have Spanish/Portuguese ancestry. Many Sephardim now live in Israel, and they constitute only a small minority of the Jewish populations in English-speaking countries.

Ashkenazim and Sephardim each have their own distinct languages, traditions, and cultural heritage, as well having different genetic conditions that predominate.

The current Jewish population worldwide is estimated to be around 13 million. Around 6 million live in the United States, and approximately 5.8 million live in Israel. In the United Kingdom, the Jewish population is estimated at around 300,000.

Religious Streams

Religious groups in the Jewish world vary according to their level of adherence to *halacha* (ha-la-cha, Jewish law) and their level of engagement with the outside world. Starting with the most religious, a simplistic description of each group follows:

Ultra-Orthodox or Charedi

The Charedi (Cha-ray-di) refer to themselves as Strictly Orthodox; this group actually comprises many smaller sects, each of which follows a specific leader/Rabbi or Rebbe (Re-bee). The most well-known term used to describe this community is Hassidic (Has-id-ic), although technically this term only applies to a certain subsection of the ultra-Orthodox world. Parts of this community are somewhat insular, and they follow Jewish law very strictly. Men and women do not interact outside of the family (aside from in work/business), gender roles are traditional, and families are large. Distinctive dress for men usually includes long black coats, various types of black hat depending on the particular sect, and the wearing of beards and side-locks (payos). Women dress modestly, and married women cover their hair with either a wig or hat (or both). Important decisions are often made with the guidance of the local Rabbi, even on intimate matters (see Box 4.1).

Box 4.1 Case Study 1: The Strictly Orthodox Client in the Genetics Clinic

On the whole, these families would be expected to attend the genetics clinic if they are referred. From the outset, it is appropriate for the clinician to be mindful of interactions between the genders. A female clinician should avoid shaking hands (or making any other physical contact) with a male ultra-Orthodox client, and vice-versa. Although some Orthodox and ultra-Orthodox clients will return a handshake from a clinician of the opposite gender (so as not to embarrass the clinician), they would feel far more comfortable if this situation did not arise.

Following from this, it is worth being aware that it will be difficult for some ultra-Orthodox clients to even make direct eye contact with a healthcare professional of the opposite gender. This lack of eye contact should not be taken as offensive to the clinician, or as a sign of hostility or avoidance of the issues at hand because it is often a result of routine segregation of the genders in this group.

If a young, unmarried, ultra-Orthodox client (whether male or female) is referred, it is very likely that he or she will attend with parents, partly because of the huge involvement of parents in their children's lives up until they are married, but also because, in this community, young people should not be alone behind a closed door with a member of the opposite sex. Theoretically, medical consultations can be exempt from this requirement, but even so it is not a situation that young ultra-Orthodox people are comfortable with.

When taking a blood sample, in which physical contact is necessary, if it is practical in the clinical setting, then it will be much appreciated if the offer is made of a clinician of the same sex to take the sample.

With regard to family dynamics in ultra-Orthodox families, it will often be the case that husbands and fathers appear to dominate in discussion with clinicians and decision making. However, as in all clinical situations, it is important for the genetic professional to attempt to include women in all discussions as much as possible.

If difficult medical or reproductive decisions are required, it would be normal for these clients to consult their own Rabbi for guidance, after the clinic. It is unlikely, although not impossible, that a Rabbi would attend the clinic with the family.

The majority of the ultra-Orthodox world speaks Yiddish as a first language, but many also speak English. It is most likely that a Yiddish-speaking family will have at least one English speaker who will act as an interpreter, if necessary. The option of an external Yiddish interpreter could also be offered prior to the consultation, but it is likely that most families would prefer to preserve their privacy by keeping interpreting within the family.

Modern Orthodox

This group follow the traditions and laws carefully but also interact more with the outside world than do the ultra-Orthodox. In this group, women also dress modestly and married women cover their hair with a hat but not usually a wig. Men in this group will usually wear a kippah (ki-pah) or yarmulke (yar-mul-ke) (both terms for skullcap) but will not wear the distinctive dress of the ultra-Orthodox.

The Modern Orthodox Client in the Genetics Clinic

In this group, many people will prefer not to have physical contact with members of the opposite sex, for instance, shaking hands. However, they would not expect a medical professional to realize this. Sometimes the easiest policy when in doubt is for a female professional not to offer a handshake to any Jewish male wearing a skullcap.

Non-Orthodox Groups

There are several streams of Judaism engaged in an attempt to further balance Jewish life with the modern world. These groups each have slightly different philosophical positions and historic backgrounds, and they all take a more flexible approach to the interpretation of halacha (Jewish law) than do Orthodox communities.

Culturally Traditional Jews

A large number of Jews in Western countries identify strongly as Jewish and may even be members of synagogues (sometimes even Orthodox synagogues), but who actually adhere to very little of Jewish law. These families usually celebrate major Jewish festivals and life events, but on a day-to-day basis live in a similar way to the majority of Western society. However, the Jewish world is highly organized and active, and many nonreligious Jews participate in activities such as cultural pursuits, voluntary work, or charitable endeavors. In this way, many Jewish people are engaged with the Jewish community without necessarily being religiously observant.

Secular Jews

A proportion of the Jewish population are completely disconnected from the Jewish religious world, although they may have varying degrees of cultural identity.

In the cases of those affiliated with non-Orthodox groups, culturally traditional Jews, or secular Jews, it would probably be fair to say that life choices and important decisions are made by the same set of criteria as others in the Western world. Halacha and Jewish tradition in general are likely to have minimal impact in areas such as reproductive decision making.

In terms of the overlap between different ethnic groups and religious streams, the majority of the diversity of non-Orthodox streams is found in the Ashkenazi world.

The Sephardi world is, on the whole, fairly conservative about its religious traditions, and the majority of its population could be described as modern Orthodox or culturally traditional, as well as having its own ultra-Orthodox sects. This does not preclude individual Sephardim from joining non-Orthodox Ashkenazi synagogues. However, liturgical traditions and synagogue customs differ between Ashkenazim and Sephardim and this may discourage Sephardim with non-Orthodox philosophies from joining Ashkenazi non-Orthodox communities.

The Changing Nature of Modern Jewish Families

Another important issue to address at this point is that the Jewish population is changing in modern times. Whereas a generation ago the Jewish population could be expected to consist of traditional nuclear families, the current population is no longer uniformly in this mould. In 2001, the question of religion was asked for the first time in a U.K. Census. This has allowed for more analysis of the U.K. Jewish population than has ever been possible before. The data have demonstrated that although around three-quarters of Jews still marry within their religion, a sizeable proportion are either married to non-Jews, co-habiting, or living in single-person households (Graham, Schmool, & Waterman 2007). The analysis of the 2011 U.K. Census will provide the first opportunity to see how these trends are changing over time, and the development of the modern Jewish community and fate of the nuclear family. It is unlikely that the Jewish community aspects of this data will be available for analysis before late 2012 (personal communication with Jonathan Boyd at the Institute of Jewish Policy Research).

Jewish Marriage and Family

Peru U'Revu
And God blessed them; and God said to them: "Be fruitful and multiply, and replenish the earth, and subdue it." (Genesis 1:28)
—Translation from the Pentateuch edited by Rabbi Dr. J. H. Hertz, 2nd edition, 1987

Be fruitful and multiply, or in biblical Hebrew "Peru u'revu," is noted in Jewish tradition as the first commandment that is made by God in the Torah (To-rah) (the five books of Moses). This divine directive has been internalized as a driving force in Jewish life. Unlike some branches of Christianity, Judaism does not ascribe holiness to celibacy, but rather to marriage and procreation. Within the Orthodox and ultra-Orthodox communities this commandment is spoken of and revered as the ultimate purpose of adult life and more specifically marriage. In this community, young people marry at younger ages than in mainstream Western society, and they have many children. The ultra-Orthodox world is set up to accommodate and support this lifestyle, and so strong is this culture that the majority of its young people follow this preordained path into adulthood without deviation. Later in this chapter, we examine in more detail the way the Orthodox world organizes and regulates these areas of life.

However even in the non-Orthodox and culturally traditional sections of the Jewish community, the importance of having children drives much of Jewish life. This often creates immense pressure for young Jews to find a spouse and start a family. The stereotype of Jewish parents and grandparents frequently asking young adults "Nu?"(Yiddish for "well?") "Have you met anyone nice?" or "When will we have grandchildren?" still exists in modern Jewish life. There is often little censorship of this expectation from one generation onto the next, and although this may be so normalized that it goes unnoticed, it can also trouble those who do not manage to fulfil it. In this part of the Jewish world, marriage and children are not subject to so many laws and customs as in the ultra-Orthodox world, but are still a primary focus of family life and held in high esteem. As a result, for young Jews who may be pursuing a college education and starting careers, the hope and assumption of this aspect of their future may be more prominent in their minds than for their non-Jewish Western peers.

The Jewish marriage ceremony is held under a "Chuppah" (choo-pah; a canopy), and the assumption of a future containing marriage (and hence, children) is so strong that the traditional blessing recited for a new baby declares the wish for this child to enter a life of "Torah (meaning a religious life), Chuppah (indicating marriage), and good deeds." This blessing is recited at the circumcision of all Jewish baby boys, the naming ceremony of Jewish baby girls, and is uniformly used across the Jewish world. So, from the day a Jewish baby enters the world, the hope that he or she will eventually marry and have children of his or her own is at the heart of Jewish tradition.

An Aside: Attitudes to Science and Medicine

And God blessed them; and God said to them: "Be fruitful and multiply, and replenish the earth, and subdue it." (Genesis 1:28).

This verse not only tells us of the importance of family to the Jewish world, but also hints at the place of science and medicine in the directive to "subdue it." The traditional Jewish attitude to science and medicine has always been one of openness, engagement, and support. This attitude stems from the tightly held belief that when God created the world, it was left unfinished and imperfect. In doing so, God chose to give human beings the opportunity and ability to improve the world.

In modern times, this imperative has led to a great tradition of Jewish doctors, scientists, and philanthropists who support science and medicine. Even within the Ultra-Orthodox world, there is far more interest and openness to developments in science and medicine than might be expected from such a traditional and closed community.

Arranged Introductions and the Emerging Importance of Genetics

In the ultra-Orthodox section of the Jewish world, young people are considered ready for marriage once they reach their late teens. These young people are segregated throughout their childhood and schooling and have little contact with each other outside of the family. Parents of teenagers take the lead in finding suitable potential partners for their children, often with the help of a third party (known as a shadchan [shad-chan] or match-maker). Much research is done by parents, in conjunction with the shadchan, to find the best match, and this may involve scouring connected communities in other countries. Once a potential partner has been identified, an introduction is arranged, and, if the couple like each other, they may "date" on a few occasions (within strict guidelines—they must never be alone together behind a closed door or touch each other) before announcing their engagement within a few weeks and marrying within a couple of months. However, it is important to note that the young people are also free to reject the match and ask their parents to look again, and so this process may go on for some time. In this way, members of the community do not define themselves as practising arranged marriages and prefer to call this process "arranged introduction" or shidduch (shid-oo-ch).

> There has always been a concern about family health history in this community, and, even before the advent of modern genetics, a family with an inherited disorder (or a disorder that was assumed to be inherited) could have trouble finding a shidduch for their children. Parents routinely ask about the family history of a potential suitor for their child and use this information in assessing suitability.

Therefore, it should not be very surprising that, in recent years, genetic screening has become an integral part of the shidduch process. This screening is specifically aimed at avoiding the genetic conditions that predominate in this population. This started solely as Tay Sachs screening but has now grown to include about ten different recessive genetic disorders. However, to avoid possible stigmatization of carriers of these diseases (and hence of their whole families), an innovative (if sometimes controversial) screening program was developed within the ultra-Orthodox community, called DorYeshorim (ye-shor-im) (Ekstein & Katzenstein 2001) (see Box 4.2).

Box 4.2 Dor Yeshorim

Dor Yeshorim (DY) works in the following way: blood samples are collected for carrier screening from young people before they enter the shidduch process, and the individual is given a PIN number. The test results are held on an international database attached only to the PIN number and date of birth of the individual (the name and address of the individual are not stored). The test results are not given out to anyone, including the person tested. However, before two young people are introduced, the shadchan will call the Dor Yeshorim database with both their PIN numbers. If the two people are both carriers of the same genetic condition, the database will automatically show that they are "incompatible" and the introduction will be avoided from the outset. However, the condition they carry will not be revealed unless the information is specifically requested by the parties concerned.

This system ensures that, at least for these conditions, prenatal diagnosis and termination of pregnancy never have to be considered by these couples. We will examine attitudes to these interventions later, but it can already be seen that their avoidance is preferred. Importantly, this system also means that a carrier of one of these conditions will usually never know that he or she is carrying anything at all; most of the time the potential match is not a carrier of the same condition and the database returns a result of "compatible."

Some additional points to bear in mind about DY. It is an international scheme: all samples are shipped to the laboratory in New York for testing and all results are held on the New York database. The names and addresses of those tested are not stored in the database, so, if an individual loses his or her PIN number, he or she will have to be retested. Once a sample enters this system, the test results will not be released to anyone (including a future genetic professional who is counseling that individual).

Finally, DY has strict rules about "double testing." If an individual already knows he or she is a carrier of one of these conditions, he or she is not permitted to be tested by DY. This prevents the database becoming, in the long term, a repository for known carriers, with known noncarriers not requiring its services. Also, the DY organization requests that individuals tested by it should not be retested subsequently for the same conditions in any other laboratory. Its main concern in this regard is to prevent people from knowing carrier results that may stigmatize them. However, there is a self-fulfilling prophesy at work here, in that the declaration by the organization that this information would cause stigma has in itself increased stigma around genetic carrier status in this community. In other (non-ultra-Orthodox) sections of the Jewish world, where carrier testing is done with good community education and genetic counseling, carrier status has not caused stigma (Zeesman, Clow, Cartier, & Scriver 1984). However, on a positive note, this program has cleverly created a way of avoiding prenatal diagnosis (PND) and termination of pregnancy (TOP) decisions for the most common conditions in a community which would be averse to these options.

In the non-Orthodox world, marriage partners are found through dating and romantic involvements, just as in the non-Jewish Western world. However, screening for the common Jewish genetic conditions is also becoming routine for non-Orthodox couples (although this may sometimes occur after marriage or in the antenatal period) through traditional genetics service, where results are given with genetic counseling where appropriate. These screening programs are now well established in North America, Israel, and Australia, although not yet available through the National Health Service (NHS) in the United Kingdom.

Population Screening for Common Recessive Conditions in the Jewish Population

In the United Kingdom, Tay Sachs screening has existed since the mid-1980s and, from 1999, it was approved by the National Screening Committee (NSC) and was given NHS funding for the laboratory and clinical costs. Tay Sachs is an autosomal recessive neurodegenerative condition that presents in infancy and causes death by the age of 4 in most cases. Jewish community groups educate about this issue, promote screening, and run community and high school screening sessions.

In the United Kingdom, Tay Sachs screening is not a fully established national program, so it is not routinely offered in antenatal care. However, if screening is requested by a Jewish client, there are a number of options for testing (e.g., via their general practitioner or local genetic service).

In the United States and Israel, it is now common to test for many other recessive conditions that are more prevalent in the Ashkenazi Jewish population. These conditions include (but are not limited to) familial dysautonomia, Canavan disease, Gaucher disease type I, Bloom syndrome, Niemann-Pick disease type A, Fanconi anaemia type C, mucolipidosis IV, cystic fibrosis (common AJ founder mutations), and glycogen storage disease 1a. However, this is an ever expanding list, with some laboratories in the United States now offering 17 genetic conditions on the AJ screening panel.

In the U.K. population, carrier screening for these other conditions is not available on the NHS for Jewish clients. There are private laboratories offering such tests, and recently a private service has been set up at Guy's Hospital in London, on a pilot basis. Jewish clients with a known family history of any of these conditions can, of course, be offered carrier testing free on the NHS. A new charity has been established called Jewish Genetic Disorders UK (JGD UK) in order to provide the community with more information and support regarding these issues.

PREPARING FOR THE CONSULTATION

Taking a Family History

Sadly, due to the effect of the Holocaust, when 6 million Jews were systematically murdered by Nazi Germany during World War II, many families cannot trace their recent history very far. Many families in Britain, North America, Israel, and other countries originated from individuals escaping the Nazis just before the Holocaust, or from sole survivors after the war whose whole extended families were wiped out.

> It is okay to ask a Jewish client about the Holocaust and whether his or her family were involved when taking a family history, and the question in itself is unlikely to cause offence. In fact, it is likely to be perceived as both knowledgeable and sensitive if a genetic counselor demonstrates an awareness and understanding about lack of family history information in a Jewish family affected by the Holocaust.

However, not every family is affected, and a sizeable Jewish population was already living in the United Kingdom before the rise of Nazism; these families were largely unaffected by it. So, it need not be assumed that every family will have been affected or that this will necessarily be a sensitive area. Also, as time goes on, fewer direct survivors are still alive and thus there is even less access to the family history of preceding generations. Conversely, the newer generations are less reliant on this aspect of their family history as their immediate predecessors were post-Holocaust.

Another issue when taking family histories is that the Jewish world is an international entity with many families having relatives in other communities around the world.

Reproductive Decision Making in the Face of Genetic Risk

Prenatal Diagnosis and Termination of Pregnancy

As is apparent from the DorYeshorim program described earlier, the ultra-Orthodox community prefers to avoid the need for prenatal diagnosis (PND) and termination of pregnancy (TOP) as much as possible. For the conditions that have been screened for, this system is indeed effective. However, members of this community carry the same risks as any other for unexpected fetal abnormalities to be discovered during pregnancy or at the birth of children and for other genetic conditions for which there will be a recurrence risk.

For Orthodox and ultra-Orthodox couples, interpretation of Jewish law (halacha) will usually be key to their decision making on these issues. Whether such a couple would opt for PND will largely depend on whether they would ultimately consider

TOP. In the Orthodox Jewish world, it would be fair to say that although there is not a blanket ban on TOP, it is reserved for extreme and specific circumstances.

The starting point in halacha for rulings on TOP comes from the following biblical passage:

And if men strive together, and hurt a woman with child, so that her fruit depart, and yet no harm follow, he shall surely be fined, according as the woman's husband shall lay upon him; and he shall pay as the judges determine. But if any harm follow, then thou shalt give life for life, eye for eye, tooth for tooth, hand for hand, foot for foot, burning for burning, wound for wound, stripe for stripe. (Exodus 21: 22–25, translation from the Pentateuch edited by Rabbi Dr. J. H. Hertz, 2nd edition 1987)

In this passage, it is clear that the fetus does not have the status of a fully fledged life, and killing it does not constitute a capital crime, as it is not covered by the later requirement of "a life for a life," and the one who causes its loss is subject only to a fine. However, this verse does not equate in halacha to permission to wilfully terminate a pregnancy for any reason.

The laws regarding requests for TOP in various scenarios are not a straightforward matter, and various biblical passages, along with the writings of ancient Sages, and past and contemporary Rabbis can all be drawn upon. These are then subject to the interpretation of local Rabbis, whose opinions may vary among communities and different Orthodox sects.

The only straightforward situation in which TOP is uniformly permissible in halacha is when the pregnancy threatens the life of the mother. In this case, it is clear in Jewish law (derived from a section in the "oral law" Mishna Ohalot 7:6) that the mother's life takes precedence. However, as might be expected, the ultra-Orthodox community tends to be less permissive of TOP for other reasons, often including fetal abnormality or genetic disorders.

However, there is a tradition in Jewish law that the fetus only acquires status as a life 40 days after conception. Before that time, the embryo is considered "mere water" (derived from the interpretation of the oral law in the Talmud, Yevamot 69b). Theoretically, attitudes toward TOP could be more lenient during this timeframe but, even then, the halacha is complex in this area. However, it has not been possible to offer PND and TOP before the 40th day of gestation; it will be interesting to see how attitudes to free fetal DNA testing develop as this technique becomes a more widely available at much earlier gestational dates.

It is no doubt the case that even within the ultra-Orthodox community there have and will continue to be instances in which couples have opted for PND and, where appropriate, TOP, despite halachic rulings to the contrary. Therefore, although generalizations can be made about the likely reaction to these issues for this population, one can never apply these as a blanket assumption to an individual member of this group. When counseling Orthodox and ultra-Orthodox couples in such situations, it is appropriate to demonstrate sensitivity to the need for Rabbinic consultation, while still making it clear that the clinician can provide information and support regarding all possible options. It is likely that a couple will listen to the options presented by the clinician and subsequently discuss these with their Rabbi. If a couple requests, it may also be appropriate for the clinician to explain these options to the Rabbi, to help the Rabbi guide the couple.

> Non-Orthodox Rabbis have been known to use a more flexible interpretation of the notion of pregnancy threatening the life of the mother and include within it the threat to the mother's psychological state and future well-being. This allows for justification of TOP for medical reasons when there is fetal abnormality or a genetic disorder.

However, in reality, few non-Orthodox Jews would feel bound by halachic rulings or even be aware of their content. For the majority of the Jewish population, these types of decisions are made based on personal moral and ethical codes. It would not occur to most non-Orthodox Jews to consult their Rabbi on a decision of this nature.

Preimplantation Genetic Diagnosis

Preimplantation genetic diagnosis (PGD) is a process whereby embryos are created using in vitro fertilization (IVF) technology and biopsied on the 3rd day to remove one or two cells. Genetic testing can then be performed on these cells to determine which embryos are affected with the genetic condition in question. Unaffected embryos can then be transferred to the woman's uterus, while affected embryos are left to perish or donated to research. Unused healthy embryos can also be frozen for use in later cycles.

As described earlier, an embryo that is less than 40 days old does not have the status of a living being in halacha. There have been complex halachic arguments over the exact status of an embryo prior to the 40th day, and also questions about the differences between an early embryo in utero versus one in vitro. Unlike an early embryo in utero, the embryo in vitro cannot become a life if it remains in its current state, therefore possible prohibitions on abortion do not apply to it. Following from this, it is permissible to discard embryos that are found through PGD to be affected with a genetic condition.

> In general, with regard to both IVF and PGD, the vast majority of contemporary halachic authorities now consider these acceptable options, even in the ultra-Orthodox world.

It goes without saying that all couples using any form of assisted reproductive technique (ART) have concerns about samples being mixed up in the laboratory. After several high-profile cases of such occurrences, there are now strict regulations in the United Kingdom (as imposed by the Human Fertilization Embryology Authority, the U.K. government body that regulates ARTs) on the labeling and witnessing of all procedures and sample transfers in embryology laboratories. However, an extra element of concern arises in Jewish law because the Jewish status of a child is determined by who his or her parents are, and aspects of this status then influence various laws on who that child can marry.

> Ultra-Orthodox couples sometimes request that a Rabbi who is knowledgeable about ART be present in the embryology laboratory to observe and give halachic verification to the status of their future children. There are now a small number of Rabbis with expertise in this area and a number of fertility clinics who are happy to work with them to facilitate halachic supervision of ART.

Gamete Donation as a Reproductive Choice to Avoid Genetic Disease

When discussing reproductive options for couples at risk of having a child affected with a genetic disorder, an often quoted option is that of *gamete donation*, using gametes that are not carriers of the disorder in question. For ultra-Orthodox couples this area could be particularly problematic, because, like some other religious groups, some halachic opinions regard sperm donation as adultery. The other concern about sperm donation is that a future child may end up in an incestuous relationship with an unknown sibling conceived using the same donor sperm.

For this reason, where sperm donation is permitted, it is often suggested that a non-Jewish sperm donor would be preferable to a Jewish one, to avoid future incest. The other problem with sperm donation is that, according to Jewish Law, the obligation to procreate falls on the man (the female partner merely facilitates his fulfilment of this obligation). Hence, using another man's sperm to have children may mean that he has not fulfilled his legal obligation (the exception to this is that, if he is azoospermic, then he cannot fulfil his obligation anyway, and it is sufficient for him to have tried).

> For these reasons sperm donation is problematic for many ultra-Orthodox couples. However, there is intense halachic debate on this matter and it would still be reasonable for a clinician to mention this option as one that the couple may wish to discuss further with their Rabbi.

Egg donation is also a complex option, although for different reasons. The issue here is that a child is only considered Jewish by virtue of having a Jewish mother. This leads to a debate over who is considered, in halacha, to be the true mother of the child—the one who gives birth or the one who supplies the genetic material—and accordingly, whether the donor must be Jewish. Again, an Orthodox couple would need to consult their Rabbi before pursuing this option further. However, in this area, even a non-Orthodox couple may have concerns about the future Jewish status of their child.

COMMUNICATION IN THE CONSULTATION

Medical Screening for Those at Increased Risk of Disease

The general approach of halacha (Jewish Law) to medicine and health is that we have an obligation to take care of our body and our health, which is God-given. We are viewed as the caretakers of our bodies, rather than the owners, and hence this is our duty. This would include preventative or precautionary measures for preserving health, such as screening to detect early signs of cancer. In fact, if anything, the cultural trend in the Jewish community is to be so overly concerned about health that Jewish clients could be perceived by medical professionals as somewhat pushy, or even neurotic!

There may be some concerns among more Orthodox clients about intimate examinations by medical professionals of the opposite gender. However, although there may be a preference for a female client to see a female doctor, there is no prohibition on seeing a male doctor. As there is always a concern among the ultra-Orthodox about being behind a closed door with a member of the opposite sex, it would be normal for a client to bring a family member as a chaperone or request a chaperone in the clinic, especially for examinations and procedures.

Death, Mourning, and Postmortem

The Jewish traditions around death and mourning are very specific. It is of utmost importance to bury the deceased as soon as possible, even on the day of death if this can be achieved, but certainly the next day or the day after at the latest. Great emphasis is placed on the concept of "respect for the dead" and the preservation of the body for burial. The body must be buried whole, with all its parts, and so postmortem examinations or autopsies are often a problem for Jewish families, both because they delay the funeral and because of the fear of the body not being buried whole. However, if a coroner orders a postmortem this would be allowed by a Rabbinic Authority, with the caveat that all histological samples should be returned for burial if possible. In the case of postmortems undertaken to make a genetic diagnosis or to advise on recurrence risk in the future, Rabbinic opinions range from full permission to those that are more stringent.

As soon as the funeral has happened, first-degree relatives of the deceased and the spouse enter a period of official mourning. This begins with 7 intense days of mourning, known as "sitting shiva" (shi-ver). The official mourners spend the days of the coming week at the home of the deceased (or sometimes at the home of another member of the family who is hosting the shiva), where they sit on low chairs and receive visitors who come to offer condolences. Prayers are also said in the home each day of the shiva. During this time, the mourners are prohibited from work and household chores.

The Jewish approach to mourning aims to gently ease the mourners from the most intense early stages of grief gradually back to normal life. After the first 7 days, the mourners enter a less intense period of mourning that lasts until the 30th day after the funeral. During this time, mourners return to work and daily life but also have certain restrictions, for instance a prohibition on participating in celebrations that involve music and dancing. The official mourning period actually lasts for a whole year, and Orthodox Jews will continue to avoid music and dancing and will say a daily memorial prayer.

ACKNOWLEDGMENTS

The author would like to thank Carolyn Cohen (Support Worker for the Jewish charity "Chana") and Rabbi Chaim Weiner (Director of the European Masorti Bet Din) for their advice, suggestions, and proofreading of this chapter.

RESOURCES

www.jewishwomenshealth.org
www.jewishgeneticdisordersuk.org
www.jlaw.com

REFERENCES

Biale, R. (1984). *Women and Jewish law*. New York: Schocken Books Inc.

Brietowitz, Y. *The pre-embryo in Halacha*. Accessed April 7, 2012 from http://www.jlaw.com/Articles/preemb.html

Freedman, B. (1999). *Duty and healing—foundations of a Jewish bioethic*. New York and London: Routledge.

Greenberg, B. (1983). *How to run a traditional Jewish household*. New York: Simon & Schuster Inc.

Klein, I. (1992). *A guide to Jewish religious practice*. New York: Ktav Publishing House Inc.

Spitzer, J. (2005). *A guide to the Orthodox Jewish way of life for healthcare professionals* (3rd ed.). London: J. Spitzer.

REFERENCES

Ekstein, J., & Katzenstein, H. (2001), The Dor Yeshorim story: Community-based carrier screening for Tay-Sachs disease. *Advances in Genetics, 44,* 297–310.

Graham, D., Schmool, M., & Waterman, S. (2007). Jews in Britain: A snapshot from the 2001 census. *Institute of Jewish Policy Research.* Accessed April 7, 2012 from http://www.jpr.org.uk/publications/publication.php?id=195

Hertz, J. H. (1987). *The Pentateuch and Haftorahs—Hebrew text, English translation and commentary* (2nd ed.). London: Soncino Press.

Zeesman, S., Clow, C. L., Cartier, L., & Scriver, C. R. (1984). A private view of heterozygosity: Eight-year follow-up study on carriers of the Tay-Sachs gene detected by high school screening in Montreal. *American Journal of Medical Genetics, 18*(4), 769–778.

5 Communicating with Clients from the Irish Traveller Community

Jacqueline Turner

The single biggest problem in communication is the illusion it has taken place
—*George Bernard Shaw*

Irish Travellers are a culturally distinct ethnic minority group with origins believed to go back as far as the 12th century (Sheehan 2000). They have their own culture, traditions, and values that set them apart from the rest of the Irish population. The accepted term and one which Travellers use to describe themselves is "Irish Traveller." They are a recognized racial group for the purposes of the U.K. Race Relations Act of 1976 and are therefore legally protected from discrimination (Diacon, Kriteman, Vine, & Yafel 2007).

Roma (Romany gypsies) are a separate legally recognized ethnic group and have their origins in nomadic tribes from northern India in the 11th century.

> Irish Travellers tend to marry within their own community and have done so for generations. Thus, certain genetic conditions are more prevalent in the Traveller population than in the "settled" (i.e., non-Traveller) community; some of these conditions are so rare that they are seen exclusively within the Traveller community.

It is common for Irish Travellers to marry members of their extended family, frequently first or second cousins. As a result, they share a proportion of their genes and are more at risk of having children with autosomal recessive conditions.

Irish Travellers are poor attenders at all outpatient appointments and in our experience often fail to attend their genetic counseling appointments. Many reasons are postulated as to why Irish Travellers may fail to attend. It may simply be that they do not fully understand the nature of the appointment and what issues are discussed in a genetics clinic.

Irish Travellers often miss out on conventional education, many having left school at a young age and having received scant education. Illiteracy is high among Irish Travellers. It is important to be aware of this when explaining difficult concepts or providing written information.

My interest in the Irish Travellers began when I became part of the Traveller Consanguinity Working Group (TCWG) (2000–2003), a group set up to address the need for a genetic counseling service for Travellers and to examine the genetic risk associated with consanguinity (see Box 5.1).

Box 5.1 Case Study

Mr. Martin Stokes and Miss Katie Stokes were referred to the clinical genetics service by their parish priest. They are first cousins and wish to get married as soon as possible, but the priest wants them to meet with a genetic counseling service to discuss health implications for their children.

An appointment was sent to the couple but they failed to attend. This was followed-up with a phone call to Katie. She did not understand why they were referred. When an explanation was provided of what was covered in a genetic counseling session, she was interested in attending and an arrangement was made to meet with her and her partner the following week.

They attended clinic and were very knowledgeable about their family history. Much of the session was spent drawing the pedigree, as Miss Stokes came from a family of 17 and Martin came from a family of 12. Most of their siblings were married with children, and all the children were healthy. Their parents also came from large families. Katie's sister was married to Martin's brother. Katie's mother and Martin's father were brother and sister. One of their cousins had two children with Down syndrome.

The genetic counselor explained that many people across the world marry their relatives and, although it is not widely practiced in Ireland generally, the genetic counselor said that she had met with many related couples from both the settled and the Traveller community to discuss the implications for their children.

Using diagrams, the genetic counselor explained genes, chromosomes, and how Katie and Martin shared half their genes with their siblings. The pedigree and the diagrams were used as a basis for explaining autosomal recessive inheritance. The genetic counselor checked for understanding throughout and in a nonthreatening manner, and asked pertinent questions to make sure the salient messages were being followed. The genetic counselor was careful to explain that, as with any distinct group, certain genetic conditions were more common and that it would be possible to test for these.

The genetic counselor carefully drew the pedigree and explained why she needed to confirm the diagnosis of Down syndrome. She also mentioned that it is unusual for someone to have two children affected with Down syndrome.

She then informed them of the general risk for consanguineous unions and offered carrier tests for galactosemia (1 in 11 carrier frequency in the Irish Traveller population). The couple readily accepted the offer of testing and blood was taken.

Following the appointment, the genetic counselor confirmed that the cousin's children have Hurler syndrome, not Down syndrome. The mutation is known, and carrier testing is possible.

The genetic counselor arranged another meeting with the couple to explain these findings. The couple were encouraged to consider how they would feel if they were both found to be carriers for Hurler syndrome and to consider what impact an unfavourable result would have on their future family planning. They both agreed to testing for Hurler syndrome. It was suggested that they discuss the possibility of an unfavorable result with each other after the counseling session so that they both were in agreement with each other. As it happened neither were carriers for Hurler syndrome. The couple indicated that they found the meeting useful and were very grateful for the information.

BACKGROUND

A comprehensive survey of Travellers has revealed that 40,129 Travellers are living on the island of Ireland today; 36,224 in the Republic of Ireland and 3,905 in Northern Ireland (All Ireland Traveller Health Survey [AITHS] 2010). Thus, Travellers form approximately 1% of the Irish population (north and south included).

The number of Irish Travellers living in mainland Britain is unknown. The British census from 2011 will be the first to officially categorize Roma and Irish Travellers as distinct ethnic groups. However, estimated figures indicate approximately 300,000 Roma and Irish Travellers in mainland Britain (Commission for Racial Equality Report into Gypsies and Irish Travellers 2006).

There appear to be pockets of Irish Travellers in the United States, each with a population of possibly a thousand or more. Again, there are no accurate figures because the U.S. census does not recognize them as a distinct ethnic minority group.

The Irish Traveller population is very bottom heavy: the Traveller Health study 2010 revealed that 63% of Travellers are under 25 years of age (compared with 35% nationally) and that 3% of Travellers are over 65 years of age (compared with 13% of the general population). This population structure is due to both high rates of fertility and premature mortality.

Although fertility rates for Travellers have come down in recent years, due to an increasing desire for family planning, the average Traveller family is still large when compared with the general population. Irish Travellers have the highest fertility rate in Europe (AITHS 2010).

Irish Travellers have a higher rate of mortality for all causes of death. Traveller males have a mortality rate 3.7 times that of the general population. Traveller male life expectancy is 61.7 years, as compared with 76.8 years in the general population. For Traveller females, the mortality rate is 3.1 times the general population, with a life expectancy of 70.1 years, compared with 81.6 years in the general population. The most common causes of death among Travellers are heart disease and stroke (32%), cancer (22%), and respiratory disease (12%) (AITHS, 2010).

Infant mortality is 3.6 times higher than in the general population (AITHS 2010). The occurrence of sudden infant death syndrome is estimated to be 12 times greater among Travellers than in the general population (McDonnell, Cullen, Kiberd, Mehanni, & Matthews 1999).

Culture

It is useful to be aware of particular aspects of Traveller culture before beginning genetic counseling, including *nomadism, intermarriage, language,* and *faith.*

Nomadism

Travellers are traditionally a nomadic group, often undertaking seasonal migrations. Nomadism has social, economic, and cultural value. Nomadism is a fundamental part of Traveller identity.

Travellers travel in closely knit nuclear families. They travel to attend larger family gatherings such as weddings, christenings, funerals, and anniversaries. These gatherings serve to strengthen family ties and to arrange meetings with marriage partners.

Today's Travellers are much less nomadic than they were in the past; many Travellers no longer travel at all, and of those who do, most travel during the summer months (AITHS 2010).

Intermarriage

Irish Travellers generally choose marriage partners from within the Traveller population. This is borne out by the fact that the Traveller genome differs from the general Irish population's genome. However, when compared with other population groups, Travellers are most closely related to the Irish general population (Dr. Sean Ennis; personal communication 2011).

Irish Travellers, like many other societies, have a history of intermarriage. Intermarriage means that marriage partners are chosen from extended family members for economic and social reasons. There is also a tradition of arranged marriage, in which parents or an elder will choose the marriage partner for a particular son or daughter.

As extended family members lose touch due to limitations of the nomadic life-style, parents have a smaller number of potential marriage partners for their children. This has led to an increase in marriage between more closely related couples (consanguineous unions) than in the past. It is estimated that between 19% and 40% of Traveller marriages are between first cousins, although there is little reliable information and these figures are likely to be an underestimate (TCWG 2003).

Irish Travellers tend to marry younger and have their children at younger ages than their counterparts in the general population. The maternal age profile of Traveller mothers has not changed since 1987. The average maternal age is 25.9 years compared with 31 for the general population (AITHS 2010).

The increase in marriage breakdowns and separations has meant that arranged marriages are not as prevalent as they were in the past, but they still may be as high as 80% for some families (Sheehan 2000; personal communication TCWG, 2002–2003).

Language

The Travelling community predominantly speaks English, but Travellers have their own language called Cant, Shelta, Gammon, or Minceirtoiree. Sometimes, Travellers will use words from their own language between themselves during a genetic counseling session.

Faith

Irish Travellers are predominantly Roman Catholics (98% in the Republic of Ireland and 96.7% in Northern Ireland) (AITHS 2010). They may have strong links to their local church and receive a lot of support from their clergy. Although many are non-practicing, most still have deep faith.

Expectant mothers usually seek a blessing for the safe delivery of their child and the health of the mother. Once born, parents normally wish for the child to be baptized as soon as possible. The age at which most Travellers marry is young and most marriages take place in church. The Catholic church requires 3 months notice of a couples intention to marry and requests that all couples attend a premarriage course.

Education

Travellers tend not to settle in one place for very long, and this tends to disrupt schooling. Policies are in place for the state to provide ethnically appropriate pre-school, primary, secondary, and senior training colleges for Travellers; however, the numbers of Travellers attending full-time education are still very low.

The 2006 census revealed that 63.5% of Traveller children under the age of 15 had left school, compared to 13.3% nationally. For these reasons, Travellers tend to have high illiteracy rates, reportedly as high as 80% (NICTP 1992). In a more recent study, difficulty reading and filling out forms was reported by 28.8% of Republic of Ireland families and 35.3% for those in Northern Ireland (AITHS 2010).

Employment

In the past, Travellers were largely based in the rural community, working as tin-smiths, seasonal farm laborers, and door-to-door salespeople. As more Travellers move into urban areas, a shift to different occupations has occurred. Travellers have become involved in the buy-and-sell trade, horse trading, scrap collecting, tarmac laying, and antique dealing. Traveller economy is based on providing services on an immediate cash basis. Unfortunately, the majority of Travellers are unemployed and dependent on social welfare payments. The 2006 census quotes an unemploy-ment rate among Travellers of 75%, compared with 9% in the general population (Central Statistics Office 2007). These figures were at a time of economic prosperity for Ireland, and unemployment is likely to have risen even higher today. Travellers feel discriminated against and believe that discrimination hinders their entry into the labor market.

Past Experience with the Medical Profession

In the past, the medical profession was generally much more paternalistic and there was less focus on good communication with clients. Therefore, some Traveller fami-lies have had bad experiences with the health service, because they resented being told what they should do. There have been instances of Traveller children being hospitalized rather than being sent home for fear of poor compliance with a spe-cific diet (TCWG discussions 2000–2003). There are reports of new mothers being encouraged not to breastfeed for fear the child may have galactosemia. Travellers do not place the same trust in the medical profession as comparable population groups (41.9% as compared with 81.8%) (AITHS 2010). Travellers report feeling that physicians make little or no attempt to explain conditions or treatment in an understandable manner.

Traveller Identity

Most Travellers are proud of their roots and will readily tell you that they are a member of the Travelling community. Others have settled into the community and may be embarrassed by their roots. They may wish to turn away from their Traveller identity because they are worried about the negative public perception of their ethnic group.

It is useful to include ethnicity, rather than nationality, as one of the standard questions at the beginning of a genetic counseling session, explaining why this information is useful and giving examples of various ethnic groups in the population. By normalizing the query, the genetic counselor will help avoid causing the Traveller client unnecessary worry about being prejudged or stigmatized.

Genetic Risk Associated with Consanguinity

Consanguinity is a favored custom across many communities in North and sub-Saharan Africa, the Middle East, and much of Asia, regions with a combined population of 720 million (Bittles 1994). It is generally not practiced across most of Western Europe. The lack of familiarity with this cultural practice can result in an exaggerated negative view of the risks of consanguineous marriage among the general population (Modell 1991).

"Health workers frequently tell consanguineous parents of children with a congenital disorder that their child is sick *because* they are related"(Modell 1991). A nonjudgmental attitude is important when dealing with communities in which consanguinity is common. It is important to be clear about the risks involved and not to overestimate them. It is also important not to blame consanguinity for a disabled child; this simply causes shame and stigmatization and is very unhelpful.

Genetic risk for consanguineous marriage is only for autosomal recessive conditions and some congenital malformations (TCWG 2003).

Degree of Relationship

The degree of homozygosity, and therefore the chance of having a child with an autosomal recessive condition, increases the more closely related a couple are. The population risk for any couple having a child with a serious congenital abnormality is 2.5%. The excess risk for a couple who are first cousins, in the absence of a known genetic disease in the family, is 3%. This excess risk is a result of autosomal recessive conditions.

Therefore, the risk of having a child with a serious congenital abnormality for an isolated first-cousin mating is estimated to be 5% (Harper 1998). This mirrors the figure quoted in the best practice guidelines published by the Consanguinity Working Group in the United States (Bennett et al. 2002).

For first-cousin matings within the Travelling community, where there has been a history of intermarriage, it is more difficult to quantify with any accuracy the degree of homozygosity and therefore the risk associated with a particular union.

Looking at this issue, the Traveller Consanguinity Working Group (TCWG) felt that, because consanguineous marriage is the cultural norm in the community, the genetic implications must be seen in context, and criticisms and efforts to disrupt traditional marriage patterns avoided.

> Individuals choosing to marry their first cousin have a legal right to do so, and healthcare professionals must respect their decision and support them by providing information in nonjudgmental manner.

Therefore, the TCWG recommended it as inappropriate to warn the entire population of their general risk but to offer carrier testing to those at high risk before marriage (when matches were arranged and the health service could be involved). In the absence of any quantitative study on the prevalence of certain genetic conditions in the Traveller population, it is difficult to assess carrier frequencies for particular conditions. With the exception of possibly galactosemia, with an estimated 1 in 11 carrier risk for Irish Travellers (Murphy et al. 1999), there does not appear to be any genetic conditions that are so widespread in the entire Traveller population to warrant population screening. In time, a panel of genetic tests for Traveller specific diseases may become available which will change the management of these cases.

It has also been observed that risk tends to be concentrated in particular families with specific genetic conditions more common in certain family groups than others (Flynn 1986). This can lead to an over- or underestimate of carrier frequency for particular Traveller families because carrier frequencies are based on disease prevalence in relation to population size, and the Traveller population may be broken down into separate genetically distinct families. This mirrors what has been reported for other consanguineous populations (Modell & Darr 2002).

In conclusion, the TCWG believes that, at present, careful examination of family history is all that is warranted and that carrier testing be organized based on this form of risk assessment (TCWG 2003). Carrier testing can be arranged for relatives before they marry and, when matches are made, this information can be taken into account. This reflects the approach made by other communities in which consanguinity is common, such as the DorYeshorim premarital genetic testing for the Ashkenazi Jewish population (see Chapter 4).

Genetic Conditions That Occur in the Irish Traveller Population

The National Center for Medical Genetics in Dublin is continually collating genetic conditions seen in the Irish Traveller population. Some of these conditions are so rare that they are seen almost exclusively in particular Traveller families, whereas other conditions occur both in the Traveller population and the settled community. Because the Traveller population is small and marries within itself, however, these more common conditions appear to be more prevalent in this population.

Irish Travellers are quite a homogeneous population from a genetic perspective (Personal communication, Dr. Sean Ennis 2011). Thus, when a condition is known, there tends to be specific mutations with the gene (founder mutations).

Classifying Risk for a Particular Family

Obtaining an accurate family history is usually relatively easy with Irish Travellers because knowledge of the family history is often extensive and accurate. Although dates of birth are not always known, names, surnames, and relationships are. However, there is often a lack of medical/scientific knowledge about particular conditions or illnesses, the names of which do not appear relevant. It is sometimes helpful to ask if there are any family members who have had problems with learning or who have attended a special school.

> Down syndrome is a label frequently applied when a child has intellectual delay, but this may not be the actual diagnosis. As with all genetic consultations, it is essential to confirm the diagnoses in the family.

> However, it can be difficult to confirm diagnoses in the Traveller community because these large families have recurring names and surnames, dates of birth may not be known, and the family may have moved a number of times since the child was born.

Dealing with Genetic Risk: Options for Pregnancy

Travellers, whether practicing or not, may still hold strong Catholic beliefs on the use of contraception and termination of pregnancy (TOP). The Roman Catholic Church bans all artificial forms of contraception, with abstinence being the only birth control allowable. The Roman Catholic Church believes that TOP is morally wrong, and it teaches that human life begins at the moment of conception. As a result, Travellers are more likely to decide that their family is complete, rather than to test a pregnancy because they would not choose to terminate an affected pregnancy (Experience of the National Center for Medical Genetics, Dublin). However, it is important not to stereotype here, and there are still many Travellers who would consider TOP. Any discussions about recessive conditions should also include a discussion of all family planning options, including preimplantation genetic diagnosis and the use of donor eggs or sperm.

PREPARING FOR A CONSULTATION

In our experience at the National Center for Medical Genetics in Dublin, Travellers are poor attenders at clinic, potential barriers to access the genetic service could be a lack of understanding regarding the reason for referral or inability to read the appointment letter. They may also wrongly assume that they will be told not to have children or that they shouldn't marry within the family. There is evidence that these fears and concerns a prevalent among other minority groups (e.g., the Deaf community; see Chapter 1). Travellers are typically referred following the birth of a child with a genetic disorder and consider the consultation to be about their risks of having a further affected child. This is usually discussed at the time of the diagnosis and may be considered irrelevant, especially if the couple has decided not to have any further children. An opportunity to discuss cascade testing may be missed, in that Travellers often miss genetic appointments.

> It is good practice to ensure that you have a phone number so that the client can be called before his or her appointment to check his or her understanding and answer any questions he or she has about the reason for the referral. When given accurate information about the purpose and potential benefits of genetic counseling, Travellers will attend appointments.

Travellers obtain most of their health-related information from their general practitioner (GP, 91.1%) (AITHS 2010). It is important that GPs be aware of the clinical genetic service and the benefits such a service has for Traveller families so that they can relay this information to their clients.

There has been a move toward enabling Travellers to provide healthcare to their own community. All regions of the Health Authority in Ireland (North and South) have a Traveller-specific health worker. Genetic services can make contact with the local Traveller health worker to liaise with a particular family.

> As family history information is of utmost importance when evaluating risks for Irish Traveller families, it is important to allow enough time, perhaps an

extra 20 minutes, to record this information during the consultation. Traveller families are large, and Irish Travellers are usually very knowledgeable about their families.

COMMUNICATION IN THE CONSULTATION

As many Travellers have received scant education and are unlikely to have a good knowledge of science, the use of visual aids is important during the genetic counseling session.

When obtaining family history information, it is important to explain why this information is necessary. Many Travellers tend to name their first son after his paternal grandfather. Thus, for large families, there may be several people with the same name. This naming custom can make it challenging to confirm a diagnosis. It is important to ask for as much information about the child as possible, his or her parents' names (including the mother's maiden name) and where they were living at the time of the diagnosis. If a child has died, it is important to ask the age of the child when he or she died. Many Irish Travellers have strong links with those who have passed on and may continue calculating their age.

The National Center for Medical Genetics in Dublin has a number of large Traveller pedigrees, thus improving the accuracy of information and ensuring that a couple is tested for all the conditions present in the family. If a Traveller family is seen by a different clinical genetic service while on their travels (e.g., within mainland Britain), it may be helpful to contact the Dublin team to find out if the family are already known to the service.

If there is no genetic condition present in either family, carrier testing for galactosemia can be offered to consanguineous Traveller couples without documented history because of the high carrier frequency in this population.

Because Travellers may not have had a conventional education, they may lack certain math skills. This needs to be considered when presenting risks as percentages or fractions. The Travellers have a long association with the horse industry, however, and may more easily understand risks presented as *odds*. For example, when explaining the risk of an affected pregnancy for a recessive condition, the genetic counselor can quote both 3:1 odds instead of a 1 in 4 risk.

Strongly held Roman Catholic beliefs may mean that discussion about TOP should be treated cautiously, and it is important to ask for views on this subject before making assumptions.

High illiteracy rates mean that the some Travellers may not be able to read. However, summary letters (which are standard following most clinical genetic consultations) are still very helpful. Even if the proband cannot read the letter, he or she still likes to receive it and will often ask a family member or other health worker to read it to him or her. Travellers may be embarrassed by their inability to read and may not be forthcoming about this. It may be helpful to explain that a summary letter is provided to everyone who attends for genetic counseling but that it is also possible to offer this in an audio format, too.

When working with the Traveller community, it is helpful to provide the family with the genetic counselor's contact details so that these can be passed on to family members. It is also useful to make a post-clinic follow-up telephone call to check if the information was understood.

SUMMARY

- Always telephone before the clinic appointment to explain the reasons for the consultation and what can be gained from a genetic consultation.
- Allow an extra 20 minutes for obtaining a detailed pedigree.
- Confirm all diagnoses and stillbirths.
- Because of their distrust of the medical profession, explain your reasons for obtaining a family history and why clarity is important.
- Be mindful that many will have received a scant education and may be illiterate; present information with diagrams whenever possible. Present risk in a number of ways; stress that the risk is per pregnancy.
- Never make a client feel that his or her child has a particular condition because the parents are related; it is nobody's fault.
- Many Travellers are Roman Catholic and may hold strong beliefs on TOP; be careful how you approach this issue.
- Provide clients with your contact details following the consultation and follow-up with a phone call to see how the information was received.

RESOURCES

http://paveepoint.iePavee Point is an Irish NGO supporting Human Rights for Irish Travellers

REFERENCES

All Ireland Traveller Health Study Team. (2010). *Summary of findings*. School of Public Health, Physiotherapy and Population Science, University College, Dublin.

Bennett, R., Motulsky, A. G., Bittles, A. H., Hudgins, L., Uhrich, S., Lochner Doyle, D., et al. (2002). Genetic counselling for consanguineous couples and their offspring:

Recommendations of the National Society of Genetic Counselors. *Journal of Genetic Counseling, 11*, 97–119.

Bittles, A. H. (1994). The role and significance of consanguinity as a demographic variable. *Population and Development Review, 20*, 561–584.

Central Statistics Office. (2007). *Census of population of Ireland 2006 place of work census anonymised records.* Cork, Ireland: Author.

Commission for Racial Equality Report into Gypsies and Irish Travellers. (2006). *Common ground: Equality, good race relations and sites for gypsies and Irish travellers.* Accessed April 6, 2012 from http://www.equalityhumanrights.com/uploaded_files/publications/easyread_gypsies_and_travellers.pdf

Diacon, D., Kriteman, H., Vine, J., & Yafel, S. (2007). *Out in the open: Providing accommodation, promoting understanding and recognising rights of gypsies and travellers.* Accessed April 6, 2012 from www.bshf.org/scripting/getpublication.cfm (accessed 6 April 2012)

Flynn, M. (1986). Mortality, morbidity and marital features of travellers in the Irish midlands. *Irish Medical Journal, 79*, 308–310.

Harper, P. S. (1998). *Practical genetic counselling* (5th ed.). Oxford, UK: Butterworth Heinemann.

McDonnell, M., Cullen, A., Kiberd, B., Mehanni, M., & Matthews, T. (1999). A national model of care service for professionals dealing with Sudden Infant Death. *Irish Journal of Medical Science, 168*(4), 237–241.

Modell, B. (1991). Social and genetic implications of customary consanguineous marriage among British Pakistanis. Report of a meeting held at the Ciba Foundation on 15th January 1991. *Journal of Medical Genetics, 28*, 720–723.

Modell, B., & Darr, A. (2002). Science and society: Genetic counselling and customary consanguineous marriage. *Nature Reviews Genetics, 3*, 225–229.

Murphy, M., McHugh, B., Tighe, O., Mayne, P., O'Neill, C., Naughten, E., & Croke, D. (1999) Genetic basis of transferase-deficient galactosaemia in Ireland and the population history of the Irish Travellers. *European Journal of Human Genetics, 7*(5);549–554.

NICTP (Northern Ireland Council for Travelling People). (1992). *With—not for, community development with travelling people.* Briefing document for ACT Conference, Belfast.

NorthernIreland Statistics and Research Agency. (2005). *Northern Ireland census (2001) key statistics.* Accessed April 6, 2012 from http://www.nisranew.nisra.gov.uk/census/pdf/ks_sett_intro.pdf

Sheehan, E. (Ed.). (2000). *Travellers: Citizens of Ireland.* Dublin: Parish of the Travelling People.

Traveller Consanguinity Working Group (TCWG). (2003). *A community genetics approach to health and consanguineous marriage in the Irish traveller community.* Position paper. Accessed April 6, 2012 from http://paveepoint.ie/travellers-and-issues/travellers-and-consanguinity/

6 Communicating with Clients from the Pakistani Muslim Community

Mushtaq Ahmed

The difference between the right word and the almost right word is the difference between lightning and the lightning bug.
—Mark Twain

The frequency of most genetic conditions among the Pakistani community is generally the same as for the general population. There is, however, an increased risk of certain autosomal recessive disorders in this population due to its high rates of consanguinity (Shaw 2003). In spite of these medical risks, there are psychosocial, social, and economic advantages to consanguineous marriages, and this is a tradition that will continue to thrive. Cousin marriages are a valued cultural tradition, a preferred practice, and integral to the structure of many societies. Consanguinity is practiced across many different parts of the world (Hamamy et al. 2011). Marriage between close relations ensures the retention of status or identity and, in some parts of the world, land and property in a family. This, in turn, serves to strengthen family ties.

According to the 2001 U.K. Census, there were 706,539 Pakistanis in England, of which 650,516 identified themselves as Muslim. Forty-three percent of all Muslims in England are Pakistani. The Pakistani population is mostly concentrated in Lancashire, Yorkshire, West Midlands, and Greater London. Greater London, as a whole, has the largest Pakistani population, but at the local authority level, Birmingham has the largest Pakistani population, followed by Bradford and Kirklees, in West Yorkshire. More than half of the Pakistani population growth since 1991 is accounted for by U.K.-born Pakistanis. In England, the city of Bradford has the largest proportion of its total population (15%) identifying themselves as of Pakistani origin. This population mostly resides in areas of high social deprivation

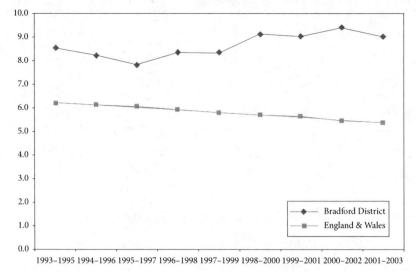

FIGURE 6.1

Infant deaths per 1,000 births, 1993–2003. Reproduced with permission of District Infant Mortality Commission.

and is associated with higher than average infant mortality (Bradford District Infant Mortality Commission [BDIMC] 2006). As with many other Pakistani populations that have immigrated to other countries, infant mortality is well above the average in Bradford (Figure 6.1).

The Bradford and District Infant Mortality Commission (BDIMC) reports that at least 25% of the deaths between the ages 0 and 12 months are attributable to congenital abnormalities. Nonmalignant life-threatening central nervous system conditions are four times more frequent in South Asian children than in indigenous white children, and 1 in 100 Pakistani babies die from lethal malformations. Consanguineous marriage is considered a risk factor for increased neonatal mortality and morbidity due to the increased prevalence of autosomal recessive conditions. It has been reported that the rate of consanguinity is high in Pakistani Muslims in United Kingdom, and this trend is increasing (Shaw 2001, 2003).

The impact of consanguinity is not only relevant to autosomal recessive conditions; Pakistani families and individuals may also seek genetic counseling to discuss autosomal dominant conditions, chromosomal abnormalities, and sex-linked conditions. Irrespective of the mode of inheritance, it is, however, not uncommon for consanguinity to be discussed in almost all counseling sessions with Pakistani clients.

BACKGROUND

This chapter focuses on communication issues that are relevant to genetic counseling for Pakistani Muslim clients. As a Pakistani Muslim myself, I draw on more than

20 years experience of working in and with this community as part of my role as a senior registered genetic counselor at the Yorkshire Regional Genetics service based in Leeds, U.K.

> Pakistani Muslims are not a homogenous group. The Pakistani community in the United Kingdom has originated from different parts of Pakistan and, therefore, may have different cultures and languages. For example, not all non-English speaking Pakistani clients speak or read Urdu, which is the national language of Pakistan.

Translation and Interpreting in Genetic Counseling

In British and U.S. multicultural societies, genetic services often provide counseling to clients whose first language is not English. A pilot study conducted in the United Kingdom found that 24% of clients from ethnic minority backgrounds indicated that English was not their preferred language for a genetic consultation (Mehta 2003).

> Pakistani clients are one of the main recipients of genetic counseling in the United Kingdom who may speak languages other than English (e.g., Urdu, Punjabi, Mirpuri, Hindko). For the majority of Pakistani couples referred for genetic counseling, at least one partner does not speak English. It is therefore the responsibility of genetic service providers to ensure that accurate genetic counseling is provided in an appropriate Pakistani language that the family or individual understands (Darr 1999).

There can be serious consequences for the Pakistani individual or family if no provision is made to provide genetic counseling in their preferred language (Anionwu 1996). For example, without accurate genetic counseling, there may be a tendency to blame women in the male-dominated Pakistani culture for the birth of a child with a genetic condition. Lack of spoken English can hinder direct communication with health professionals (Middleton, Robson, Burnell, & Ahmed 2007). Although it is acknowledged that cross-cultural differences warrant equitable and effective genetic services (Clarke & Parsons 1997; Penchaszadeh 2001; Shaw 2003; Weil 2001), there has been very little discussion and assessment of interpreting and translation provision in genetic counseling (Shaw & Ahmed 2004).

Pakistani languages lack equivalent terms that are used in genetic counseling. It can therefore be a challenge to convey correct concepts in a target Pakistani language.

> Even some of the common, everyday words used in genetic counseling do not have direct translations in Urdu (e.g., "cousin," "aunt," and "uncle"). Similarly, some genetic terms, such as "gene," "chromosome," and "recessive inheritance,"

have technical meanings that lack direct equivalents in Pakistani languages (for details, see Shaw & Ahmed 2004).

Shaw and Ahmed (2004) have described a number of problems inherent to the use of translated educational materials in genetics; for example, "recessive" was translated into "subdued" or "out of sight," "tests during pregnancy" became "pregnancy tests," "genetic counselor" translated as "expert in procreation" and "carrier" as "sufferer." Shaw and Ahmed (2004) concluded that it is appropriate to retain some of the genetic terms in English rather than attempt to translate them into Urdu (see Box 6.1).

Some genetic services in the United Kingdom employ bilingual Pakistani genetic counselors to counsel Pakistani clients, whereas others may need to arrange qualified interpreters. Some genetic counselors may not use professional interpreters due to the lack of resources or availability of interpreters in a target language. It is not uncommon to use family members, including children, as interpreters, which may have ethical, medical, and psychosocial implications. Also, when relying on English-speaking relatives, it is impossible to guarantee that accurate information is passed on to clients (Shaw 2003). Some of the recommendations from Box 6.1 can be used for face-to-face consultations with the help of qualified interpreters.

As always when using interpreters, it is important to provide them with full information about the consultation prior to its delivery. This allows the interpreter to prepare for certain phrases and concepts and ensures that he or she has had the chance to rehearse and check meanings. However, it is important to not reveal too much personal information about the client ahead of the consultation—the interpreter should not know private medical information before the client is informed, and, if bad news is to be broken, the interpreter should not know the result ahead of the client. Having said that, the interpreter should

---

Box 6.1 Recommendations for Translating Genetic Leaflets

- Practice close collaboration between bilingual professionals and translators.
- Encourage freedom to use words and phrases of target language.
- Practice minimal use of technical terms and give no unnecessary information.
- Make sure technical terms are explained clearly in everyday words and phrases.
- Encourage the freedom to change and improve English text.
- Provide dual-language text, including glossary terms and explanations.
- Test communication by piloting with target population.
- Use back-translation from Urdu into written English to double-check accuracy. From Shaw & Ahmed 2004.

be warned that there is the possibility that a range of information will be delivered, some of which may be emotionally difficult for the client—forewarning of this is imperative.

Similar to recommendations for translation, interpreters should be given the freedom to use appropriate words and terms from the target language to explain genetic information. However, genetic counselors should aim to discuss this with the interpreter first, so that they can clarify that the closest meanings are used.

Pakistani Muslim Names

In the clinical genetics service, it is important to understand the naming system of particular client groups, especially those that may not fit with the European naming system (e.g., Pakistani Muslim names).

Lack of understanding of such systems may lead to incorrect names being recorded on the genetic database. This, in turn, can result in multiple entries of the same client on the system; difficulty in locating the correct client; and genetic clinic appointments and post-clinic letters going to the wrong people and thus creating potential breaches of confidentiality. To avoid confusion and offence, it is important that both administrative and clinical staff have training about nontraditional naming systems. Once understood, most Pakistani names fit easily into the European naming system. Pakistani Muslim names are discussed in Boxes 6.2 and 6.3.

Box 6.2 Pakistani Names

In most Pakistani families, the last name is not shared within the family and each member has a different surname.

- Husband—Mohammed Ali
- Wife—Razia Begum
- Sons—Mohammed Khan and Saleem Ali
- Daughters—Parveen Bibi and Fatima Bi

Pakistani Male Names

Male names can consist of two or three parts (first, middle, and last name or surname). The last part can be a family/surname. A personal or "calling name" can be either the first or second name. In the following examples, the underlined name is a male "calling name," and these are informally used by family or friends. Health professionals can ask clients for their preference and how they would like to be addressed both informally and formally. There are no set rules for addressing Pakistani men informally for calling names (as, for example, in European system, where the first name is used as a calling name), and these can be either first, second, or the last part of the full name.

For example:

- Mohammed Hussain
- Ali Amir Qureshi

Male names can be hyphenated and, as such, can be difficult to record on a genetic database. In the following two names, "Hassan" and "Din" can be used as surnames for the recording system; the underlined name can be used to address Pakistani men, informally.

- Zia-ul-Hassan
- Ghulam-ud-Din

The first or second part of a male name may be a religious name. Extreme care should be taken when addressing a client in person or in a letter so as not to mix up the religious name. If religious names are separated out, offence can be caused.

- Allah Ditta ("Allah" means God and "Ditta" means given; thus, "God Given," e.g., a child born after many unsuccessful attempts at conception)
- Allah Rakha ("Allah" means God and "Rakha" means protected or saved; thus, "Saved by God," e.g., a child born and survived after many miscarriages or neonatal deaths)

How to address a Pakistani male?

- Formally, by title and full name (e.g., Mr. Mohammed Hussain).
- Informally, by either full name or calling name; this can be checked with the client, as either the first or second name can be the informal calling name (e.g., Mohammed Hussain)

How to record a Pakistani male name?

- Obtain a full name (usually two, occasionally three parts).
- Enter the last part as a surname (e.g., Full name: Mohammed Hussain;
- Surname: Hussain)
  (Do not assume that that Mohammed Hussain's wife's surname will be Hussain.)

PREPARING FOR THE CONSULTATION

In an ideal world, every consultation with a Pakistani client would be delivered in a culturally and linguistically sensitive manner (Darr 1999). Unfortunately, this isn't always the case. Consultations are often inaccessible to Pakistani clients, and this can

Box 6.3 Pakistani Female Names

Pakistani females usually have two-part names. The first name is a personal or calling name. The second name is often not shared with the family. The second name is usually a female title (e.g., Bi, Bibi, Begum, Kauser, and Jan). If the second name is not a female titles, it can also be a calling name.

- Amina Begum, Fatima Bi, SaleemaBibi

How to address a Pakistani female?

- Formally, by title plus full name (e.g., Mrs. Amina Bibi)
- Informally, by full name or calling name (usually the first part; e.g., Amina Bibi)
- In letters, by full name (e.g., Amina Begum)
- In a letter to couple, Mr. Full Name and Mrs. Full Name (e.g., Mr. Mohammed Ali and Mrs. Fatima Bi)
- In a letter to parents, Parents of + Full Name of the Child (e.g., to the Parents of Mohammed Khan)

Do not call Amina Bibi Mrs. Bibi; she is called Mrs. Amina Bibi.
How to record female names?

- Obtain full name (usually two parts).
- Enter the last name as surname.
  - Full name: Amina Bibi
  - Surname: Bibi

(Amina Bibi's husband will not be Mr. Bibi, as Bibi is a female title.)

have serious consequences (Anionwu 1996). It may be difficult to get the correct family history, and this may lead to incorrect diagnoses. Clients may not be able to understand critical information or inform others in the family about possible risks and may in turn not take up available services. Clinical genetic services that have a significant ethnic minority client group, such as those from Pakistan, should train and employ a linguistically and culturally matched genetic counselor to work specifically with this group. Within the United Kingdom, such genetic counselors are employed at the Yorkshire Regional Clinical Genetics Service, the Leicester Genetics Service, and the West Midlands Regional Genetics Service (see Box 6.4).

As discussed earlier, it is very important to use correct names in appointment letters, and staff who book clinics should be instructed to give the right level of attention to this. Care should be taken to ensure that, if the appointment is for a child, his or her name is correct and it is the parents who are invited to attend (i.e., the letter should not be addressed to the child). It is not uncommon for Pakistani Muslims to choose religious and hyphenated names for their children. These can often have

> **Box 6.4** The Clinic Booking Process
>
> When clients receive an invitation to attend a clinic appointment and are asked to confirm that they can attend this appointment, it is common for Pakistani clients to not respond. Irrespective of a lack of spoken or read English, they may be culturally not used to doing this. Therefore, to confirm that a clinic letter has been received and that the client intends to come, it is useful to employ the services of a bilingual or multilingual member of the appointment staff to contact clients by telephone. This definitely reduces the "fail to attend" rate.
>
> It is also important to take into account certain days and times when Muslim clients may not be able to attend clinic appointments (e.g., on the days of religious festivals and at mid-day on Friday, as it is a special prayer time).
>
> Clinic attendance during the month of Ramadan is often low. Ramadan is the 9th month of the Islamic calendar, in which Muslim fast from dawn to sunset. The dates of Ramadan vary, moving backward by about 10 days each year depending on the cycle of the moon. Information about the Islamic calendar and festivals (including other religions) is easily available on the Internet. Low attendance during the month of Ramadan does not mean that clients will not attend during this month, but it may be a reason why some prefer not to. It is therefore worth confirming with clients whether they will attend their appointment beforehand.

special connotations or meanings. For example, if a couple has a baby boy after a number of miscarriages, they may call that baby "Allah Rakha" ("Allah" means God and "Rakha" means saved or protected); "Rakha" is not a name. It is an Urdu word. Together with "Allah," this gives a meaning or explanation. In this case, the couple believes that the child has been saved or has survived by the will of God. Unlike other names, this name cannot be separated. Therefore, in an appointment letter, we should avoid the salutation: "Dear parents of Allah" or "Dear parents of Rakha." The matter can be made even worse if the baby Allah Rakha died after birth and the appointment letter went out to "Dear parents of Allah" or "parents of Rakha." In Islamic belief, Allah (God) has no parents and no children, and Allah cannot die. To avoid this, in the absence of parents' names, the best practice would be to address the parents as just "parents of Allah Rakha" in the appointment letter (i.e., the name is not split up, there is no salutation, and thus no inference of parental names is made).

Cancellation of a Clinic Appointment

Caution should be heeded when a client cancels his or her clinical genetics appointment and requests not to be seen again. This is particularly the case when the referral letter clearly suggests the benefit of genetic counseling for the family. Efforts should be made to clarify the reasons for canceling the appointment or for not wishing to be seen.

Box 6.5 Case Study 1

A young Pakistani couple was referred because of the recent diagnosis of cystic fibrosis (CF) in their daughter. Their daughter's pediatrician asked the couple if they would like to have genetic counseling. The male partner could speak English, whereas the wife could not. He asked his wife whether they should see a counselor. The wife said no. Despite this, the pediatrician referred them for genetic counseling. When they received the appointment letter, they wanted to cancel their appointment and said they did not wish to be seen. The appointment officer (an administrative member of the staff who books appointments) informed the Pakistani genetic counselor about the couple's decision. The Pakistani genetic counselor telephoned and discussed the situation with the couple. They thought that they were being offered therapeutic counseling when said they were coping well with the diagnosis of their daughter. The genetic counselor explained what genetic counseling was and the purpose for seeing the couple. The genetic counselor subsequently met the couple. The couple very much appreciated the effort that had been made to explain why they might like to come to the clinic, and also really appreciated the information they learned from genetic counseling.

It turned out that the couple were very isolated within their extended family. The mother blamed herself for her daughter's condition and therefore avoided discussing CF. Once, she understood the inheritance of CF and its implications, she started transferring information to other relevant family members. She felt empowered and, in turn, facilitated decision making about carrier testing for herself, her husband, and other members.

The reason may be that the client is not aware why he or she was referred or had some misconceptions about counseling, as illustrated in the example in Box 6.5. It is therefore important that a proactive but sensitive approach be used in these situations.

COMMUNICATION IN THE CONSULTATION

Because the Pakistani Muslim naming system is very complicated, it is preferable to use full names when calling clients from the waiting to consultation room. It is not uncommon for Pakistani Muslims to miss their appointments because the wrong name has been called. Using incorrect names can be offensive for Muslim clients, as discussed earlier. Once clients are in the consultation room, how they would prefer to be addressed can be clarified.

It is important to avoid shaking hands with clients, particularly with clients of the opposite sex, unless offered. It is both culturally and religiously offensive and thus not offering to shake hand with clients is considered polite.

Before starting the consultation, the genetic professional needs to establish who is present. It is common practice for Pakistani Muslim clients to be accompanied by their relatives, friends, and sometimes neighbors, for a number of reasons (e.g., they were driven to the hospital, need assistance with language, or need someone to look after the children they brought to the consultation with them).

Pakistani clients are often unaware of what information will be discussed during a genetic consultation. They may not want to share information with neighbors or acquaintances about the risks of having further affected children or the implications for their children's children. Disclosure of such information can ostracize parents of affected children and can also jeopardize their children's future marriages, as they may be considered coming from a "problem family." Therefore, it is vital to offer some forewarning that very personal information will be discussed; it may also be important to take the lead and say that another appointment will be booked for them to come back—this is because simply asking the client in front of the neighbor or accompanying relative if it is appropriate for them to stay will not suffice. Clients will often be too polite to refuse and will not wish to appear rude to their companion. If the genetic counselor does not pick up any unease about this, there is a high chance that the client will suffer in silence and shame as his or her personal information is discussed. It is very important to be sensitive to this issue and take the lead in arranging another appointment, even though this action might appear rather directive. It is possible to say to the client, "In this appointment, we will take some basic information about your history and then we will arrange another appointment for you to come back on your own. It is our policy to see parents on their own (thus absolving the client of any responsibility about making this decision)."

Similarly, it should also be ascertained what language the client would prefer for the consultation and, once this is known, then appropriate provisions should be made. Pakistani Muslims use a number of different languages or dialects of the same language. It is important that care is offered in the language required, as it is an essential component of service provision (Middleton, Ahmed, & Levene 2005). Genetic counselors should also not assume that any client wearing traditional dress is unable to speak English.

As with other types of consultation that cross culture and language, it may be appropriate to extend the time needed for the consultation, particularly if an interpreter is used. The length of the consultation may vary depending on whether the interpreting is being conducted by a Pakistani genetic counselor who is co-counseling with an English-speaking colleague, or whether the consultation is conducted entirely using an external interpreter. A joint session consisting of co-counseling between a Pakistani genetic counselor and an English-speaking geneticist and a Pakistani client may need an additional 15 minutes to adequately explain concepts in two different languages.

A consultation conducted using an independent, external interpreter who facilitates a conversation between an English-speaking genetic counselor and a Pakistani client may need an additional half hour, so that accurate translation can be achieved, with frequent checks for understanding. The consultation using the Pakistani genetic counselor will be quicker because he or she already has a good understanding of how to translate genetic terminology into various Pakistani languages. An external interpreter may not have this skill, and thus interpretation may take longer for him or her.

External interpreters are often limited in their experience of working with complex genetic data, and this must be taken into account. The target language of the client may lack appropriate words to interpret or translate genetic terms. I have witnessed consultations in which interpreters have struggled to communicate adequately. Interpreters are trained to translate information word by word, which may not be possible if the target language lacks linguistic equivalence. It is therefore essential to discuss such issues with the interpreter prior to consultation. The interpreter should be told that it is acceptable to use the same genetic terms in the target language rather than to look for an equivalent word to explain the concept.

> It is acceptable not to translate the term "chromosome," but to use the English word, because there is no equivalent word in Urdu. I have seen an inexperienced interpreter translate "chromosome" as "worm," probably because chromosomes look like worms! The client was told they had "worms in their blood"! A more culturally meaningful description would be to compare a chromosome to the rosary prayer bead (that Muslims use to count their prayers). Counting along the rosary beads could be a metaphor for counting along the genes structured on a chromosome.

Some terms can be translated into Urdu; for example, the word "cell" is translated as "Khuliya" in Urdu. This is not an everyday term, so only people with good educational backgrounds would understand it. Such a word should therefore be avoided. Instead, English-language genetic terms like "cell," "chromosome," and "gene" should be used directly, since it is likely that Pakistani individuals have heard these terms already via the media and also through meetings with other health professionals.

> For convenience or when there is a lack of resources, the temptation is often to use hospital administrative staff or family members (including young children) as interpreters. Genetic counseling is a difficult process, and relying on untrained people to convey difficult information should be avoided. It can compromise care and confidentiality and can also impact the psychosocial well-being of the client. It is unethical to rely on young children and family members for communication with individuals and families in genetic counseling.

The two case studies in Boxes 6.6 and 6.7 will illustrate some of the points discussed regarding interpreting.

Box 6.6 Case Study 2

A Pakistani Muslim mother told genetic counselor about her experience with a pediatrician over her daughter's diagnosis of a disorder of sex development (DSD) (the term "intersex" was used with the mother at the time) due to congenital adrenal hyperplasia (CAH). While in the labor ward, she was told that she had to wait for the confirmation of the sex of her baby. She was told that it was not clear as to whether her baby was a boy or a girl. She was stunned by this news. She was also emotionally wounded by the manner in which this information was communicated—behind the curtains in a busy hospital ward, where other Pakistani women were also present and could hear the news. The mother felt intense shame, fearing that her close-knit Pakistani community would gossip about her daughter and their misfortune before she had even come to terms with what was happening.

The mother had a follow-up appointment to discuss the diagnosis in more detail. For this appointment, the doctor arranged to have an interpreter present. However, the mother was not asked if she wanted an interpreter and, in fact, she could speak and understand English perfectly well. When the mother was brought into the consultation room, she was introduced to the interpreter. The mother was shocked to see that the interpreter was simply a member of hospital staff who happened to speak Urdu (she wasn't a trained interpreter). She knew this was because the interpreter was actually a distant relative. The mother was embarrassed and, because the woman was a relative, she found it culturally unacceptable to ask her to leave the room. The diagnosis of CAH and its implications were discussed in the presence of the relative, and the mother felt shame and disbelief—but, most of all, she did not want her relative to know any of this private information. The mother said that she could not remember a single word from the consultation.

Commentary

The handling of this case by well-meaning but inadvertently thoughtless health professionals has had a profound impact on this mother. Whether the relative did indeed share the confidential information she learned in the consultation is unknown, but what is important is that the mother's autonomy was severely compromised and there have been enormous psychological consequences for her. First, when she was unable to announce to her family, after the birth of her baby, as to whether it was a boy or a girl, she had to deal with the perceived suspicious reaction from relatives and the community. Second, the inappropriate communication support in her follow-up appointment meant that she was not able to receive any information that she needed about CAH. Her fears and worries about the Pakistani community's reaction to her child were further exacerbated by her very real worries that inappropriate information would be shared by the interpreter. Using a hospital staff member simply because

(continued)

Box 6.6 (*continued*)

he or she speaks a particular language is inappropriate; trained interpreters follow a strict ethical code of conduct and never breach confidentiality. It is not known if this member of hospital staff had any such training or if the pediatrician checked his or her qualifications.

As a consequence of this history, when the mother came for genetic counseling, she was profoundly scarred; not only had she developed a fear of hospitals and a distrust of medical staff, but she had also developed a real fear of talking about her child.

Box 6.7 Case Study 3

A Pakistani man attended the genetic clinic with his wife and sister-in-law to discuss his diagnosis of being a balanced chromosomal translocation carrier. The consultation was delivered via co-counseling with an English-speaking consultant geneticist and a Pakistani genetic counselor. The man's wife had arranged for her sister to join them in the consultation to act as interpreter. This was unnecessary, since the Pakistani counselor was able to interpret when necessary. It transpired that the wife actually wanted her sister to be present to hear what was said in the consultation; however, her husband did not appear to be complicit with this.

The man was diagnosed as being a balanced translocation carrier following the couple's unsuccessful attempts to conceive naturally over a number of years. Both the man and his wife appeared to have very limited spoken English, but he kept insisting that he could understand English and thus wanted the consultation in English. Despite this, he did not ask any questions when his diagnosis was discussed as a possible cause of his fertility problem, and he remained very quiet and subdued. The genetic counselor tried to draw him out by communicating with him in his native language, but the man kept saying he wanted the consultation in English.

After the consultation, both the consultant geneticist and the genetic counselor reflected on the session and agreed that the genetic counselor would make a follow-up telephone call to the man. When they spoke (in Urdu), the man said that he did not understand much of the English discussion. He explained that the reason he had felt so uncomfortable was because of the presence of his sister-in-law. He felt mortified that issues around his fertility and his inability to impregnate his wife were being discussed so openly in front of his sister-in-law. Perhaps by insisting on ensuring the discussion was in English, this went some way toward distancing himself from this shame.

Who should have been the priority for the consultation? Although it was the man who had been referred, the reason for the referral was infertility, which had a direct impact on his wife. Thus, the consultation was actually delivered to the two of them as a couple. It was the wife's decision to bring her sister, under the guise of being an interpreter. Perhaps what she really wanted was her own personal support? The genetic counselor decided to start over. He arranged a new appointment for the man to attend genetic counseling on his own, to discuss the genetic basis for his infertility. He then arranged to see the couple together (without the sister). For both consultations, the sessions were delivered in Urdu, not English.

This case reminds us that clients do not always attend genetic counseling with a united agenda and that, to facilitate good communication, we sometimes have to "read between the lines" to unravel what is most appropriate for the client.

Family History and Consanguinity

Pakistani clients are often very apprehensive about discussing their family history. Some believe that there is a "campaign" against their culture (waged by the dominant White culture), and they fear that their preferred practice of consanguinity is a target.

> Pakistani parents of children affected with a genetic disorder are often told that the genetic condition in their child has occurred because the parents are first cousins (Middleton et al. 2007). It should be noted that medical conditions don't occur because of marriage choice, but because of recessive genes (i.e., a different emphasis is needed to take the blame away from the marriage). Reinforcing this misconception can negatively impact the clients' trust in healthcare professionals and services (Middleton et al. 2007).

It is very common during the genetic consultation for Pakistani Muslim clients to become defensive when talking about their family's medical history. They often mention examples of their siblings, friends, and other families (who practiced consanguinity) whose children have no genetic abnormality. It is common to believe that intermarriage has no impact on health, and couples may become defensive if they believe they are being blamed or targeted unfairly. As consanguinity is highly favored among Pakistani Muslim people (Darr 1997), discussion of this topic needs to be handled with sensitivity during the consultation. It has been suggested that genetic counselors need to be aware of genetic risk and social and cultural norms, but must respond to clients as individuals, without any assumptions (Shaw 2003). Opinions differ about consanguinity; some believe that people should be discouraged from marrying cousins (Hamamy et al. 2011; Shaw 2003) and warned of the possible risks of consanguinity. Others highlight the benefits of such a custom and believe that discouraging clients and informing them of the genetic risk of cousin marriages may alienate them from using genetic services (Hamamy et al. 2011; Shaw 2003). Shaw and Hurst (2008) reported that clients can be wary of seeking genetic advice for fear of being blamed for the birth of an affected child. It is therefore recommended that health professionals avoid using any language that may be construed as stigmatizing consanguinity, to ensure equitable access to genetic services (Shaw 2003; Shaw & Hurst 2008). Every effort should be made to reassure clients that the purpose of taking a family history and asking questions about consanguinity does not mean that they are being blamed for the family genetic condition. It is sometimes helpful to explain clearly that the purpose of drawing a pedigree is to help to understand the inheritance pattern of the condition and also to make or confirm a diagnosis. It is often easy to explain inheritance patterns to clients once the family tree is drawn. At this point, clients can be given a detailed explanation as to why consanguinity may be of relevance to their particular situation. A common lay belief among the Pakistani population is that family members share the same blood (irrespective of whether they are actually related or not). This example can be used to introduce the concept of a gene that is shared and passed down from generation to generation.

Given the sensitivity of the subject, it is important that consanguinity is discussed initially with both parents of an affected child. They should be given an explanation and information about recurrence risk and implications for other members of the family. The extended family can then become involved, and an invitation to come to the clinic can be made to them via the parents of the affected child.

Discussion of Reproductive Options

Certain reproductive options are forbidden in Islam (e.g., the use of donor sperm or eggs, or the use of a surrogate mother) since procreation is conducted only through marriage (Haleem 1993; Hewitt 1998; Ismail & Serour 1997). Termination of pregnancy (TOP) for social reasons is also not allowed in Islam, unless there is a threat to the mother's life. In some Muslim countries, including Pakistan, religious scholars have agreed on the consensus verdict (Fatwa) that it is permissible to terminate a pregnancy within 120 days of gestation for serious medical conditions. This consensus has reassured some couples who were initially hesitant to use prenatal diagnosis for thalassemia (Ahmed, Saleem, & Sultana 2000). The research evidence shows, however, that there is little knowledge of the view that Islam permits TOP for serious or fatal abnormality within 120 days (Ahmed et al. 2000; Shaw 2011) and that some practicing Muslims could not distinguish between "religious or traditional or cultural beliefs" (Ahmed et al. 2000).

Making a decision about the seriousness of a particular condition is difficult and can be subjective; thus, it is not uncommon for Pakistani Muslim couples to choose to terminate a pregnancy for a whole range of conditions (and not just those that are lethal). For example, Pakistani Muslims request prenatal diagnosis and terminate pregnancies affected by congenital adrenal hyperplasia, which is a medically and surgically treatable condition.

When it comes to discussion about reproductive options during a consultation, it is important for the genetic counselor not to assume that Pakistani Muslim couples will not accept certain options. Health professionals have often wrongly assumed that Pakistani Muslim clients will not consider a termination of pregnancy (Modell et al. 2000; Sandall, Grellier, Ahmed, & Savage 2001). Pakistani Muslims should be given exactly the same information about reproductive options as would be given to any other client group. The genetic counselor needs to play a facilitative and support role and help clients to make informed decision.

> While discussing reproductive options, the counselor should be aware that Pakistani clients often expect health professionals to be directive (Moazam 2000) and seem to be unaware of the concept of client-centered counseling and nondirectiveness (Middleton et al. 2007). Therefore, the genetic counselor should be explicit and clarify that emphasis will be placed on supporting and facilitating decision making rather than giving advice (Middleton et al. 2007).

Carrier Testing for At-Risk Family Members

The majority of recessive genetic conditions in Pakistani Muslims are extremely rare in other populations. If a mutation is known in a family, carrier testing should be facilitated, particularly if the family has a strong preference for cousin marriages. Instead of alienating clients by inferring that they shouldn't marry a cousin, it is a better to offer the option of carrier testing, so people at risk can make informed decisions about choosing a partner (who may be a cousin) and know of the reproductive options that may be available to them.

Ahmed et al. (2002) carried out a study to look at the behavior, knowledge, and attitudes of British Pakistani adults toward carrier testing for thalassemia. They found that knowledge of what it means to be a carrier, as well as the mechanics of the inheritance of thalassemia, was low and that fewer than half of the relatives of someone with thalassemia had had carrier testing (Ahmed et al. 2004). Since thalassemia is a relatively common disorder in this population, it is likely that the lack of knowledge and understanding about other, rarer, autosomal recessive conditions will be even greater. It is therefore important that genetic counselors are aware of such issues and pay particular attention to educating clients, acknowledge that it is difficult to pass information on to others, and make clear that help is available via the clinical genetics service to support dissemination of information to at-risk individuals.

Directive Versus Nondirective Counseling

Not everyone wants to make healthcare decisions about their own health (Deber, Kraetschmer, & Irvine 1996; Mazur & Hickam 1997; McKinstry 2000; Robinson & Thomson 2001), and Pakistani clients particularly prefer health professionals to tell them what to do (Moazam 2000). This outlook can be at odds with the nondirective approach adopted by genetic counselors. It is therefore quite a skill to enable Pakistani clients to engage with a nondirective model so that they can weigh up what they want to do. Evidence from other fields of healthcare shows that clients from many other cultures place less emphasis on autonomy (Bowman & Hui 2000; Jafarey & Farooqui 2005), and the family plays a more pivotal role in healthcare decisions. Furthermore, the literature indicates that people from minority ethnic groups are less likely to be actively engaged in decision making (Blackhall, Murphy, Frank, Michel, & Azen 1995; Cooper-Patrick et al. 1999) and that those individuals born in the United Kingdom but raised in a particular cultural milieu and those who are recent migrants may not value the Western model of informed choice (Ahmed, Atkin, Hewison, & Green 2004). Differences in values about informed choice may complicate and potentially interfere with care in cross-cultural healthcare encounters (Elliott 2001; Ruhnke et al. 2000). To improve communication and the quality of care, a greater understanding of the different cultural values attached to the concept of informed choice is essential for genetic counselors practicing in multi-ethnic populations largely guided by Western ethical principles (Bowman & Hui 2000; Elliott 2001). It is important that genetic counselors acknowledge these cross-cultural differences (and perhaps even name these differences with the client) and encourage clients to try to engage with autonomous decision making.

Decision Making in an Extended Family System

Pakistani culture is a family-oriented and shared culture. It is not uncommon for Pakistani clients attending genetic counseling clinics to live with their extended family. Therefore, genetic counselors will meet with clients who bring their large family to the genetic clinics with them. Clients often ask their relatives for help in decision making. This can particularly happen in the prenatal/genetic clinic, where young women attend with their older female relatives. (Pakistani men usually won't attend with their pregnant wives. These men believe that issues related to a pregnancy should be dealt with only by women in the family, often not realizing the complex nature of decision making during pregnancy.) The autonomy of young women is often compromised in these situations, particularly, if a woman has recently arrived from Pakistan to settle with her husband, and has no or very little English. Mothers-in-law of young pregnant women may use their own personal life experiences to influence decisions about the termination of an affected pregnancy. For example, a mother-in-law who may have terminated a few pregnancies for social reasons in the past may try to dissuade the young woman from terminating the affected pregnancy to compensate for her own perceived wrong decisions. The decision making process is very complex in an extended Pakistani family; there may be positive outcomes from this, in which the client is supported in making an informed decision, and there may be negative outcomes, in which the client is coerced into making a decision that doesn't fit with what he or she wants. It is very important for genetic counselors to

Box 6.8 Case Study 4

A 16-year-old Pakistani girl from a highly consanguineous family was seen by a Pakistani genetic counselor. She was told by her sister, who had a child with a recessive condition, to discuss carrier testing. The girl was very keen to have carrier testing for the known family mutation because she had decided that she would marry one of her first cousins from Pakistan. She wanted to marry a first cousin because cousin marriages in her family were more successful than were marriages from outside the family. She was aware that if she was found to be carrier and she married her cousin, there would be a risk that her future children could be affected by the recessive condition, if her husband was also a carrier. Genetic testing showed she was a carrier. She decided that she would come back to the genetics service before or after her marriage for carrier testing for her partner. After 6 years, when she completed her degree, she contacted the genetics service and requested carrier testing for her cousin husband, who recently arrived from Pakistan. The same genetic counselor met the couple to discuss carrier testing, the implications if the husband was also a carrier, and their reproductive options. If both partners were carriers, they said, they would take up the option of prenatal diagnosis and terminate the affected pregnancy. The husband was tested for the family mutation and found not to be a carrier. In this case, the genetic counselor supported the decision made at age 16, and the clients came back after having made their own informed decision.

acknowledge these differences in decision making in different cultures and, at the same time, make sure that the client's autonomy is not compromised. To facilitate this, it may be helpful to offer multiple appointments, perhaps with the couple on their own to start with (encouraging the husband to attend, even if, culturally, he is not sure it is his place) and then begin to involve others (see Box 6.8).

Religious Beliefs

In Muslim culture, there is a strong belief that God controls every aspect of an individual's life. At the same time, when facing a medical problem, Muslims also believe that it is their duty to seek help and therefore doctors and medical care are considered important (Ebrahim 2001). Therefore, it is not surprising in Muslim culture that, when problems occur, individuals seek medical help while still believing that everything is due to God's will (Haleem 1993; Sandall et al. 2001). It is also not uncommon for Pakistani Muslims to share that they have been seeking spiritual guidance and support for their family's genetic condition. It is very important to acknowledge and respect such beliefs but, at the same time, the genetic counselor should also emphasize the importance of seeking medical help for genetic conditions. For example, for some genetic conditions, medical intervention is available, and it is important that parents comply with medical treatment for their affected children, regardless of their beliefs.

Psychosocial Issues in Genetic Counseling

Despite a strong fatalistic belief, genetic conditions can have a huge psychosocial impact on Pakistani families, particularly on women, who may suffer more than men from the burden of the family condition and may also be blamed for the birth of an affected child (Middleton et al. 2007). This can further be exacerbated if women are not able to communicate in English. A lack of information in a native language can therefore have serious consequences for families (Anionwu 1996). Lack of ability to speak English not only hinders communication with health professionals, but also between couples and within the family as well, leading to misconceptions and mis-understanding (Middleton et al. 2007). For example, a non-English speaking client may rely too heavily on an English-speaking partner for information concerning the couple. It is important that the genetic counselor provides a space where clients can discuss their psychosocial issues and are supported appropriately. For example, if a female partner is solely blamed for the recessive condition, equal contribution from both parents should be emphasized.

Post-Clinic Letters

It is good practice to write a post-clinic information letter to all clients of genetic counseling. However, particular attention is needed when writing to Pakistani Muslim families. It is important to check first as to whether this is appropriate. Clients may feel apprehensive about such a letter, especially if they are living with an extended family and do not wish to share their personal information. If clients decide against receiving a letter, they should be provided with an informative leaflet about their family condition that they can take home with them after the clinic. Such a leaflet can be kept private, to be used as a reference for the clients who attended clinic, or it can be shared widely with other rela-tives. If Pakistani clients want a letter, genetic counselors should make sure it is addressed correctly, using the full names (first name + second name/surname). This will avoid the letter being opened by other family members who may share the same surname.

It may not be feasible to translate every post-clinic letter for Pakistani clients into their preferred language and dialect, and it is unnecessary to do this—although Pakistani clients may speak a particular language, they may not read it. Also, there are copious problems with the translation of written material on genetic into Urdu, as discussed earlier. What is helpful, however, is to create a set of good-quality standard information leaflets in various languages that have been back-translated, checked, and validated as accurate. These can be on common informational categories covered within genetic counseling (e.g., on certain conditions or inheritance patterns). These should always be available for the face-to-face appointment.

SUMMARY

This chapter discussed some of the issues that genetic counselors may encounter in their clinical practice when working with Pakistani Muslim clients. The chapter has also provided some suggestions that may help with genetic counseling practice for this group.

- A client may have expectations that the genetic counselor will be directive in his or her approach and give advice. Genetic counselors should introduce the concept of nondirectiveness and help Pakistani clients engage with autonomous decision making (without coercion from anyone, including extended family). ·
- The issue of translation and interpreting in genetic counseling and how this should be addressed is important.
- The Pakistani naming system is complex, and it is vital to record the names and address clients appropriately, both in verbal and written communication.
- A client may have feelings of guilt and blame due to perceived pressures from non-Pakistani communities in relation to the practice of consanguinity. It is very important that genetic counselors acknowledge that the issue of consanguinity can be a very sensitive one, and they should take care not to appear to blame consanguinity for ill health.

REFERENCES

Ahmed, S., Atkin, K., Hewison, J., & Green, J. M. (2004). *Antenatal haemoglobinopathy screening: The role of faith and religion.* NHS Sickle Cell and Thalassaemia Programme Report 2004. London: NHS.

Ahmed, S., Bekker, H., & Hewison, J. (2002). Thalassaemia carrier testing in Pakistani adults: behaviour, knowledge and attitudes. *Community Genetics, 5*(2),120–127.

Ahmed, S., Saleem, M., & Sultana, N. (2000). Prenatal diagnosis of beta-thalassaemia in Pakistan: Experience in a Muslim country. *Prenatal Diagnosis, 20,* 378–383. Anionwu EN. (1996). Ethnic origin of sickle cell and thalassaemia counsellor: Does it matter? In D. Kelleher & S. Hillier (Eds.), *Researching cultural differences in health* (pp. 160–189). London: Routledge.

Blackhall, L. J., Murphy, S. T., Frank, G., Michel, V., & Azen, S. (1995). Ethnicity and attitudes toward patient autonomy. *Journal of the American Medical Association, 274*(10), 820–825.

Bowman, K. W., & Hui, E. C. (2000). Bioethics for clinicians: 20 Chinese bioethics. *Canadian Medical Association Journal, 163*(11), 1481–1485.

Bradford District Infant Mortality Commission. (2006). *Summary report.* Bradford, UK: Author.

Clarke, A., & Parsons, E. (1997). *Culture, kinship and genes: Towards cross-cultural genetics.* London: Macmillan.

Cooper-Patrick, L., Gallo, J. J., Gonzales, J. J., Vu, H. T., Powe, N. R., Nelson, C., et al. (1999). Race, gender, and partnership in the patient-physician relationship. *Journal of the American Medical Association, 282*(6), 583–589.

Darr, A. (1999). *Access to genetic services by ethnic minority population: A pilot study.* London: Genetic Interest Group.

Deber, R. B., Kraetschmer, N., & Irvine, J. (1996). What role do patients wish to play in treatment decision making? *Archives of Internal Medicine, 156*(13),1414–1420.

Ebrahim, A. F. M. (2001). *Abortion, birth control and surrogate parenting: An Islamic perspective.* Burr Ridge, IL: American Trust Publications.

Elliott, A. C. (2001). Health care ethics: Cultural relativity of autonomy. *Journal of Transcultural Nursing, 12*(4), 326–330.

Haleem, M. A. S. A. (1993). Medical ethics in Islam. In A. Grubb (Ed.), *Choices and decision in healthcare* (pp. 1–20). Chichester, UK: John Wiley and Son.

Hamamy, H., Antonarakis, S. E., Cavalli-Sforza, L. L., et al. (2011). Consanguineous marriages, pearls and perils. Geneva International Consanguinity Workshop Report. *Genetics Medicine, 13*(9), 841–847.

Hewitt, I. (1998). *What does Islam say?* (3rd ed.). London: The Muslim Educational Trust.

Ismail, M. S., & Serour, G. I. (1997). Assisted reproductive medicine: Current Islamic biomedical rules. *The European Journal of Contraceptive and Reproductive Healthcare, 2*(3), 161–165.

Jafarey, A. M., & Farooqui, A. (2005). Informed consent in the Pakistani milieu: The physician's perspective. *Journal of Medical Ethics, 31*(2), 93–96.

Mazur, D. J., & Hickam, D. H. (1997). The influence of physician explanations on patient preferences about future health-care states. *Medical Decision Making,17*(1), 56–60.

McKinstry, B. (2000). Do patients wish to be involved in decision making in the consultation? A cross sectional survey with video vignettes. *British Medical Journal, 321*(7265), 867–871.

Mehta, P. (2003). *Ethnic monitoring in clinical genetics. Project report.* London: Genetic Interest Group.

Middleton, A., Ahmed, M., & Levene, S. (2005). Tailoring genetic information and services to clients' culture, knowledge and language level. *Nursing Standard, 20*(2), 52–56.

Middleton, A., Robson, F., Burnell, L., & Ahmed, M. (2007). Providing a transcultural genetic counselling service in the UK. *Journal of Genetic Counseling,16*(5), 567–582.

Moazam, F. (2000). Families, patients and physicians in medical decision making: A Pakistani perspectives. *Hasting Centre Report, 30*(6), 28–37.

Modell, B., Harris, R., Lane, B., Khan, M., Darlison, M., Petrou, M., et al. (2000). Informed choice in genetic screening for thalassaemia during pregnancy: Audit from a national confidential enquiry. *British Medical Journal, 320*, 337–341.

Penchaszadeh, V. B. (2001). Genetic counseling issues in Latinos. *Genetic Testing and Molecular Biomarkers, 5*(3), 193–200.

Robinson, A., &Thomson, R. (2001). Variability in patient preferences for participating in medical decision making: implication for the use of decision support tools. *Quality Health Care, 10*(Suppl. 1), i 34–i38.

Ruhnke, G. W., Wilson, S. R., Akamatsu, T., Kinoue, T., Takashima, Y., Goldstein, M. K., et al. (2000). Ethical decision making and patient autonomy: A comparison of physicians and patients in Japan and the United States. *Chest, 118*(4),1172–1182.

Sandall, J., Grellier, R., Ahmed, S., & Savage, W. (2001). *Women's access, knowledge and beliefs around prenatal screening in East London. Final report*. St. Bartholomew School of Nursing and Midwifery. London: City University.

Shaw, A. (2000). *Kinship and continuity: Pakistani families in Britain*. Amsterdam: Harwood Academic Publishers.

Shaw, A. (2001). Kinship, cultural preference and immigration: Consanguineous marriage among British Pakistanis. *Journal of the Royal Anthropological Institute, 7*, 315–334.

Shaw, A. (2003). Genetic counselling for Pakistani and Bangladeshi origin Muslim families in Britain. In *The encyclopaedia of the human genome*. London: Nature Publishing Group.

Shaw, A. (2011). They say Islam has a solution for everything, so why are there no guidelines for this? Ethical dilemmas associated with the birth and death of infants with fetal abnormalities from a small sample of Pakistani Muslim in Britain. *Bioethics, 73*(1), 111–120.

Shaw, A., & Ahmed, M. (2004). Translating genetics leaflets into languages other than English: Lesson from an assessment of Urdu materials. *Journal of Genetic Counseling, 13*(4), 321–342.

Shaw, A., & Hurst, J. A. (2008). 'I don't see any point in telling them': Attitudes to sharing genetic information in the family and carrier testing of relatives among British Pakistani adults referred to a genetics clinic. *Ethnicity and Health, 3*, 1–20. doi: 10.1080/13557850 802071140URL,http://dx.doi.org/

Weil, J. (2001). Multicultural education and genetic counselling. *Clinical Genetics, 59*, 143–149.

FURTHER READING

Shaw A (2009) *Negotiating Risk: British Pakistani Experiences of Genetics*. Oxford: Berghahn Books.

7 Communicating with Clients Who Disclose Sexual Abuse

Alan Phillips

The most important thing in communication is hearing what isn't being said.
—*Peter F. Drucker*

Despite advances in the understanding of childhood sexual abuse as a form of traumatic stress, its sequelae, and treatment, much is still unknown about the subject. The false memory debacle that emerged in the 1980s (how the experience of sexual abuse is processed, encoded in memory, remembered, retrieved, relived, repressed, or forgotten) has become one of the most controversial and fiercely disputed issues in contemporary psychology (Brewin 2003; McNally 2003; Rothschild 2000; Sabbagh 2009; Yule 2003).

Studies on sexual abuse reveal a spectrum of possibilities along a continuum of traumatic stress that is influenced by a number of complex biopsychosocial variables including the type, degree, and duration of the abuse; the age at which it occurred, and the context in which it took place. One of the most enduring forms of traumatic stress, posttraumatic stress disorder (PTSD), includes developmentally inappropriate sexual experiences with or without violence, threatened violence, or actual injury and symptoms, which can equally involve "excruciatingly vivid memories of trauma" or the "inability to remember parts of the trauma" (American Psychiatric Association [APA] DSM-IV 1994).

Although every act of sexual abuse constitutes a violation of the child, and by definition renders him or her a victim, it is argued that the subtlety of some acts and/or the age at which the abuse happen, will render the experience beyond the victim's perception. Consequently, he or she will live life free of any memories and symptoms (Sabbagh 2009).

Conversely, because all the senses may be implicated in traumatic memory: taste, touch, sight, sound, and smell, others argue that, however subtle the act and even where abuse occurs at the preverbal stage of development, the person will remain susceptible to recollections of it, no matter how long after the event, as all that is needed is the right trigger or cue to reactivate the memory.

Some experiences are considered so traumatic that the only way the child can cope with the experience is through the unconscious mechanism of repression, which results in a form of amnesia. In these cases, the memories of trauma may lie dormant until reactivated by triggers or cues that are reminiscent of the original event (Courtois 1999; Frederickson 1992; Rothschild 2000).

What we learn from the various discourses is that no single definition of childhood sexual abuse, as a form of traumatic stress, exists with which to conclusively encompass all the phenomena and potential permutations involved. This presents a number of implications for adult clients, which we explore in this chapter.

The case study in Box 7.1 illustrates some of the complex permutations along a continuum of recall with which the adult client may present for genetic counseling. Where the client is on the trauma spectrum, the practitioner's knowledge of

---

Box 7.1 Case Study 1

Laura (the client's preferred pseudonym) presented for genetic counseling after many years in therapy working through her experiences of systematic sexual and emotional abuse by both parents. She had reached the point at which most of her symptoms had abated, and she was a highly functioning professional with a strong, assertive personality. Enabled by therapy, she confronted her parents, who denied the allegations. As a consequence of this, she was completely rejected by them and her extended family members who, ignorant of the abuse, were encouraged to view her as "mad," "bad," "unbalanced," "unreliable," or "untruthful." At the age of 37, she was informed by a relative that her mother was dying of breast cancer, and her father blamed her for causing it due to the stress of her "lies." Following her mother's death, Laura discovered that her maternal grandmother had also died of breast cancer, and she was advised to consider genetic testing. She describes the implications for her of attending genetic counseling as follows:

The experience of seeking advice and ongoing testing was extremely traumatic due to the fact that I was sexually abused by both parents from the age of about 11years, it may have happened earlier but I do not recollect. The memories were deeply buried and only surfaced in flashbacks etc., in my early 30s, which triggered a major breakdown. The effects of the abuse meant I could not even be registered with a new GP or dentist when I moved house 20 years ago, and, for many years,

(*continued*)

Box 7.1 (continued)

I was afraid of being sectioned under the Mental Health Act. This made me highly anxious in any medical setting but particularly with an issue that was so closely connected to my mother. For many years, I was phobic about being in contact with doctors, due to the fear of being touched or having a loss of autonomy in relation to their power. I could not tolerate anyone wearing clinical clothing or white jackets as I felt a sense of powerlessness and feared I would have no control over how I was touched or what was done to me.

Laura recalls fainting once when visiting a friend in the hospital, and, because injections or blood tests were impossible to contemplate, she concluded that "if ever I needed hospital treatment I would probably end my own life."

Ultimately, faced with the possibility of carrying the gene from which her mother and maternal grandmother had died, Laura had to confront the dilemma of whether to seek genetic testing. Although she was terrified, she knew it made sense and concluded she had had enough therapy to proceed. However, she describes how at her first consultation with a genetic counselor

...discussing the fact that my mother could have passed the gene to me made me intensely angry at her again—this time, for having given me the gene, and I went into a full physical trauma reaction. Although the counselor was empathic, I made it very brief because discussing the issue was too stressful and I realised I wouldn't be able to comply with all the requests.

Typically, Laura needed to have as much control over her environment as possible and complete control over what happened to her body:

...to sit in a gown in a public, cubicled area not knowing who was going to walk in was intolerable. Through therapy, I learned that in order to prevent the worst symptoms, I had to get into a safe zone in my head to protect myself and do relaxation exercises and cognitive work to gain a sense of ownership over my body and procedures.

As the following experience illustrates, things which would go unnoticed by an untraumatized person can trigger memories that may have a devastating effect on the survivor of childhood sexual abuse:

I once observed a father helping his young daughter remove her top clothes in a clinic (quite appropriately), and I had a full blown panic attack....

During the two month wait for her second appointment, her trauma resurfaced in flashbacks, panic attacks, and nightmares that she found "almost unbearable" and that were compounded in the consultation when:

...the anger surfaced again because the counselor assumed that it was only my father who was the abuser. It was very distressing to explain the facts. This was

(continued)

Box 7.1 (continued)

made worse because the counselor asked if another member of staff could sit in on the session. I can't recall whether it was a consultant or a colleague, but this was highly inappropriate given the content I was revealing.

The experience severely undermined any trust and confidence she had in the content, processes, and interactions involved in genetic counseling, and she concluded:

There is no guarantee of safety to a deeply traumatised individual but this could and should have been avoided...it s'aid to me that they obviously had no understanding of what I had been through and what I needed.

Although Laura accepted that in a busy hospital it would be impossible to control the environment for every potential trigger, she felt too retraumatized to proceed with diagnostic or predictive testing in this setting. Unable to tolerate the thought of attending publicly supported clinics, she opted for annual mammograms under private health care. Laura particularly appreciated her new provider's willingness to give her as much time as she wanted to disclose the abuse, associated phobias, and her needs. Like many survivors of sexual abuse, Laura is severely claustrophobic, and the mammogram procedure can activate this. As a preventative against panic attacks, Laura is allowed time to prepare for the procedure in an unrushed environment where she can apply techniques she has learned in therapy before contemplating the intervention itself. To limit the anxiety of waiting for results, which can trigger flashbacks, panic, and dissociative symptoms, she is given the results by the consultant radiologist on the same day. To prevent any reoccurrence of her previous experience, the practitioner also agreed that all this information could be included in her notes so that any subsequent professionals would be aware of her particular situation:

...this means the fact that I am a survivor of abuse is on my records and if asked why things are done differently for me, or I become anxious, I just have to refer them to my notes. This removes the need for me to repeat the story time and again. It also means I am not asked inappropriate questions and inappropriate requests are not made of me.

the subject and how they conceptualize it, and their confidence and competence to work with such clients, all have implications for the adult client presenting for genetic counseling. Against this background, the guidance offered here is informed by my work as a counselor, psychotherapist, clinical supervisor, and educator, with experience of working with clients across a broad spectrum of trauma. As the head of a multidisciplinary team of counselors and psychotherapists and as a consultative supervisor to genetic counselors and other healthcare professionals, my work regularly brings me into contact with practitioners who are faced with the dilemmas, occupational hazards, and treatment traps associated with adult survivors of sexual abuse. I am particularly grateful to the client and supervisee in the following case studies, who have allowed me to use their experiences to highlight some of the key implications and learning points for safe, effective, practice with this client population.

Reflective Commentary

The case study in Box 7.2 features an example of an adult who presented for genetic counseling with full knowledge of her childhood sexual and emotional abuse. This case study reveals how the human brain, mind, and body have very complex and

---

Box 7.2 Case Study 2

The following excerpts from a genetic counselor's supervision notes illustrate some of the dilemmas, occupational hazards, and treatment traps associated with working with adult survivors of childhood sexual abuse. These must be avoided for the health and well-being of client and practitioner alike. The client, a 45-year-old woman (who will be called Susan) attended her third genetic counseling session in a very distressed state and disclosed childhood sexual abuse, perpetrated over many years by her father, paternal uncle, and brother. This was the first time she had told anyone about it as, threatened with physical violence by the perpetrators to keep the abuse a secret, Susan had been inculcated in the belief that no one would believe her and that she would be punished for being a "dirty little girl." With a brother in prison for a serious physical assault, Susan had very real fears for her safety and that of her children, whom she does not allow her father to have unsupervised contact with. As the counselor recalls:

I felt that I had missed all the signals with this case, or perhaps was unconsciously ignoring them, which resulted in the relationship moving away from genetic issues...

Also, the appointment was time-limited and was now running over. I needed to pick up my children from school, and my mind was racing in panic. I brought the session to a very unsatisfactory end and felt that I was leaving Susan high and dry following her disclosure...

Although I lacked the specialist therapeutic counseling skills to deal appropriately with the disclosure, I hopefully did no harm. I do worry about the impact the disclosure session had on her as it must have taken immense courage to tell her story. With her consent, I referred Susan to the local mental health team for specialized therapeutic intervention. However, I realized that an appointment would take time to arrange so offered to see her again myself...

(continued)

However, by seeing Susan again, I soon discovered that she blurred the boundaries of what I was able to offer, and she began to see me more as a therapeutic counselor rather than genetic counselor. I felt that she had developed a growing dependency on me, and I soon realized that she felt reluctant to engage with the external support agency I had referred her to. However, she did give her consent for me to share the issues relating to her disclosure with the agency counselor...

I felt out of my depth and out of control with Susan's case. I wanted to try to contain it, but it felt like a car freewheeling downhill—I couldn't seem to steer the situation in any way—it felt like she was very much in the driving seat...

I had become very aware early on in my relationship with her that she bore a striking resemblance to my mother-in-law, who had died some years ago. Even her smell was similar, which was a mixture of cigarettes and air freshener...

A common theme that rears its head in supervision is my need to be liked and the anxiety that ensues. I had had a challenging relationship with my mother-in-law, who told me from the start that she did not like me, and my supervisor explored transference and countertransference [which] explained why I felt driven to help her [and] why I had allowed my patient to take the lead in the appointments as a form of overcompensation.

Follow up appointment:

I discussed the case with her external counselor, who would be seeing her, and she said that the patient must have felt safe disclosing her story to me. When we last met, she said she was finding the therapeutic counseling very helpful.

interdependent mechanisms for dealing with traumatic stress. It also exemplifies how PTSD may exist as a lifelong condition requiring specialist therapy on an intermittent, rather than one-off or constant basis (Malone 1996; Wilson & Keane 2004), during which time the likelihood exists that the person may be exposed to a number of reactivating agents such as found in medical settings. We saw how any number of seemingly innocuous cues and triggers can reactivate traumatic memories and symptoms, and, because this can have the effect on the person of reliving the experience, optimum management of the environment and the content, processes, and interactions involved can feel like a life-or-death necessity to the severely traumatized person. It is an excellent illustration of the constellation of phobias and panic, mood, and anxiety disorders associated with posttraumatic stress, the main hallmarks of which include:

- *Reexperiencing.* This includes the stimulation of any unwanted intrusions into consciousness, including flashbacks, which may be so vivid that the person feels as if he or she is reliving the actual event.
- *Avoidance.* This is characterized by the various tactics and mechanisms the person employs to minimize distress immediately following or many years after the event. Victims of trauma develop complex and creative ways of consciously and unconsciously preempting the distress of recall, including a repertoire of implicit and explicit "don't go there" messages that may be communicated as unresponsive and hostile to the well-meaning helper.
- *Ruminating.* This describes a form of cognitive intrusion typified by unwanted thoughts and the unbidden replay of exaggerated or catastrophic daydreaming and imagining that is highly resistant to rational thinking and reality testing.
- *Hyperarousal.* Worry, fear, anxiety, panic, and a sense of threat and vulnerability may prevail in the face of objective data to the contrary, leading to different degrees of hyperarousal in the form of thoughts, feelings, and physical symptoms that, in extreme circumstances, may lead to collapse.

Reflective Commentary

This case study in Box 7.2 illustrates a situation in which something in the environment and/or practitioner provided certain conditions within which the client felt safe enough, or compelled, to confide her history of childhood sexual abuse for the first time in her life. It also reveals how this can be psychologically demanding for the unsuspecting practitioner and, in highlighting some of the occupational hazards and treatment traps associated with work with this client population, provides a number of useful insights and caveats.

Transference and Countertransference: A False Connection

Susan's scenario confirms Courtois' (1999) observation that, "particular forms of transference and counter transference are likely to emerge in the treatment of traumatized/sexually abused individuals that simultaneously challenge and inform the clinician and that must be acknowledged and monitored."

The phenomena of transference and countertransference may be triggered by people, places, situations, sounds, and, as exemplified in this scenario, the practitioner's countertransference was activated by the clien's appearance and smells. It also shows how, in the context of a helping relationship, a client can project (transfer) on to the practitioner either negative or positive attributes belonging to some past significant other in the client's life. This can result in the practitioner being viewed as, and related to, as if he or she were a good, bad, or idealized mother, father, brother, sister, or other surrogate figure.

When the unconscious deficits, memories, wishes, fears, needs, or desires of the client are transferred onto the practitioner, and something in this encounter also triggers certain unconscious deficits, memories, wishes, fears, needs, or desires in the practitioner, then the unaware professional may respond by countertransferring these feelings back onto the client, thus setting up a ricochet effect of transferential messages and relational dynamics (Wilson & Lindy 1994). The case study in Box 7.2 confirms Spinelli's caveat that, as a "false connection," countertransference should always be treated as "any disruption of the therapist's constant attentive attitude" (Spinelli 2009), which, in the context of genetic counseling, should be protected against for the well-being of client and practitioner alike. As Weil (2000) points out, if left unaddressed the anxiety and discomfort that countertransference may engender in the practitioner may affect his or her clinical judgement and lead to "the avoidance of issues or to collusion with the counselee's defenses against the frightening possibility of a medically positive result."

Co-dependency and the Unhealthy Drama Triangle

No practitioner can prevent transference in their clients but the case in Box 7.2 illustrates how quickly a client's need to be nurtured and a practitioner's deep-rooted need for approval can set in train the unhealthy dynamics of a co-dependent relationship that can blur the boundaries of the legitimate, clinical remit.

As an aspect of the shadow side of helping, as Page (1999) cautions, "the intimacy offered in the counseling relationship can develop an addictive quality" that may result in an intensity of feeling that raises the vulnerability of both parties. As a form of emotional enmeshment, overinvolvement or compulsive caring, Karpman's (1968) "drama triangle," describes how the covert and unconscious roles of "victim," "rescuer," and "perpetrator" are played out in various dysfunctional ways that invariably create confusion, inhibit effective helping, and may result in serious harm (Berne 1968; Kreger 2008).

The potential for this was exemplified through the phenomenon of ambivalence, in which Susan's genetic counselor, as "wounded healer," was simultaneously attracted to and repelled by her "wounded client." As Evans (2006) suggests, the work involved in medical genetic and the countertransference issues that arise within it can make genetic counseling an emotionally challenging profession. Through judicious use of supervision, Susan's genetic counselor was able to rectify some of the treatment traps she had fallen into, bring the relationship to a satisfactory conclusion, and thus avoid some very serious consequences. However, this is not always the case. Just as survivors of trauma vary in their vulnerability to post-traumatic stress, so do clinicians whose work with trauma victims has identified them as being particularly susceptible to burnout, compassion fatigue, and even

PTSD, which can arise from their exposure to the images and narratives associated with their client's traumatic experiences and even as a result of reading material such as notes and case histories (APA DSM-IV 1994; McCann & Pearlman 1990; McNally 2003; Rothschild 2006).

Do No Harm: Establishing a Healthy Psychological Contract

As we saw in Laura's case (Box 7.1), her perceived lack of trust, confidence, and safety in the environment, content, processes, and interactions involved in her genetic counseling experience retraumatized her and triggered a range of strong emotions and behaviors including anger, rejection, and withdrawal. Conversely, something in Susan's experience led her to disclose her past abuse, for the first time, to her genetic counselor. Both scenarios reveal how a healthy psychological contract between client and practitioner is particularly important for work with the survivors of childhood sexual abuse. When children are sexually abused, the implicit, normative assumption they hold—that no harm will be done to them by their parents and other trusted adults—is significantly breached, and the more severe and more prolonged the trauma, the more negative and far reaching the effects are likely to be (Green 2004). As Cozolino (2002) suggests, the psychosocial trauma that occurs during childhood sexual abuse at the hands of caretakers and other adults makes it a "state of mind, brain and body" around which all subsequent relationships coalesce. Thus, in seeking to do no harm, the practitioner's primary responsibility is to provide the optimum conditions for trust, confidence, and safety in the environment and working alliance. The two case studies show how threats of physical assault and abandonment, along with the inculcation of fear, shame, and guilt, are common ploys utilized by perpetrators of sexual abuse to maintain control over the child and secrecy over the act.

> People who have been abused as children may have particular difficulty in trusting others and, when looking for a person to trust, continuity of care, consistency, reliability, and predictability are some of the key qualities they consciously and unconsciously seek in practitioners (Clarkson 2009; Kinchin 2005; Rothschild 2000; Scott 2008). To these ends, serious consideration should be given to how realistic, containable, and sustainable the client's expectations are likely to be within the parameters and constraints of the genetic counseling remit and the practitioner's ability to meet them.

Ensuring Safety Outside and Inside the Consultation

Upon disclosing suicidal ideation and other thoughts of self-harm, Susan's practitioner wisely sought advice from her organization's mental health team and the availability of a specialist community agency. As Laura's story illustrates, whole families may turn against the victim of childhood sexual abuse, and, in Susan's case, it shows the importance of ensuring safety outside the session, as well as in it when there is a history of violence or threats of violence and the abuser remains a potential threat to the client. Both cases indicate that it cannot be assumed that the client will be supported by his or her extended family network. The case studies illustrate how when working with families, practitioners temporarily take on the role of family member by proxy and in so doing, the genetic counselor may by necessity, become the keeper of family secrets with all the personal and professional responsibilities this entails. As well as the client's safety from reprisal of disclosure, consideration of protection and safeguarding issues regarding any children who may be at risk must be made if the abuser is still in the family or its orbit, and extreme caution should be exercised over the taking, storing, and sharing of family histories.

Fear of Compassion

One of the most counterintuitive consequences of a survivor's need to be heard and understood as part of his or her recovery may be his or her fear of compassion. In such cases, even the most empathic, nondirective, client-centered process may activate the adult client's highly attuned fight, flight, or freeze survival mechanisms, so that even when the practitioner behaves in a kind and compassionate way, which stimulates the client's innate desire for care, the feelings may be so associated with fear that the client is compelled to reject kindness (Gilbert 2009).

As a form of protective or compensatory rejection, this may not always be benign, and the professional helper may represent "the first legitimate target who will sit still and not retaliate" (Clarkson 2009). We will never know to what extent Laura's anger toward and rejection of her genetic counselor was a reflection of the residual anger she felt toward her mother. However, this can be disturbing to practitioners who are motivated to work in the helping professions and/or who are insufficiently equipped to deal with the strong, negative, or rejecting emotions and behaviors of their clients. The key here is not to take it personally but to see it as symptomatic of the client's abusive history.

Braking and Accelerating

As Rothschild (2000) observes, "you never really know how a client will react to an intervention, or, for that matter, to a simple question, the colour of your shirt, or the smell of your coffee." Therefore, the primary goal must be to contain and reduce the client's potential hypera rousal. Susan's genetic counselor's experience of being out of control and like a car "freewheeling downhill" alerts us to the need to be able to brake as well as accelerate when working with trauma victims. So that they do no harm, when taking a client's history or conducting a clinical intervention, the practitioner must have the confidence and competence to prevent retraumatization or reactivation of the client's symptoms by containing his or her reactions at any stage of the consultation or procedure. They can do this by ascertaining, or remaining vigilant for, any triggers that may lead to reactivation of the client's memories or acceleration of his or her symptoms. The well-meaning practitioner must be aware that even in trauma therapy, not all clients benefit from work with specific memories, and some even become worse; therefore, the practitioner should always tend toward braking rather than accelerating.

Using the Client's Defences as Resources

One of the simplest ways to do this is to reframe client reactions by bearing in mind that all behaviour has survival value to that individual and in this way regard the client's defence mechanisms as resources to be utilized rather than ignoring, discounting, or fighting against them. As in Laura's case, the easiest way to ensure safe practice and do no harm is to adopt the principle that the client is the best expert on what works for him or her and ask him or her what he or she needs to feel safe and secure and what you should do in the event of a trauma reaction. If you ask a client the right questions, in the right way, and at the right time, he or she will usually be able to tell you during and after each session what works for him or her and what does not.

> The genetic counseling consultation is not an appropriate forum in which to address a client's defences or coping mechanisms. Therefore, never minimize or disregard your client's coping strategies; instead, help them to create more choices within the prevailing context and setting (Rothschild 2000). Do this by adapting the consultation to the client, rather than expecting the client to adapt to it, and always respect the client's preferences. This may require the practitioner to be considerably more flexible than the usual service allows, and he or she may also need to reconsider his or her usual repertoires for handling the content, process, and interactions involved in a consultation.

AVOIDING FALSE MEMORY SYNDROME

As genetic counselors, there is no way of knowing if Laura's or Susan's experiences of childhood sexual abuse actually happened or not. Similarly, there is no reason to disbelieve or discredit their recollections of it. However, the "false memory wars" that emerged in the United States in the 1980s alerted practitioners to how highly impressionable the human psyche is to the influences and suggestions of professionals and the precautions that must be taken to avoid this (McNally 2003; Sabbagh 2009). The controversy revolves around three main issues: "(1) whether traumatic memories can be forgotten and remembered again; (2) the accuracy and credibility of recollections of childhood sexual abuse; and (3) the role of therapeutic influence on memories" (Courtois 1999). Because of well-meaning practitioners whose inappropriate interventions resulted in false accusations of abuse and led to the breakup of families and the prosecution and imprisonment of family members, professionals, and others who may have been innocent of the crimes they were accused of, false memory syndrome has been described as "the worst catastrophe to befall the mental health field since the lobotomy era" (Sabaggh 2009).

Distinguishing Between Delayed Memory and False Memory

The false memory debacle alerts practitioners to the important distinctions between delayed memory and false memory. As McNally (2003) cautions: "failing to think about something is not the same as being unable to remember it. Not having something come to mind for a period of time is not the same as having amnesia for the experience." Research suggests that memory and imagination are cued, and both rely on connections and associations to stimulate recall or imaginings. For this reason, practitioners are cautioned to be aware of how particularly potent and suggestive the cues and probes they use to elicit information can be with susceptible and suggestible clients (Sabbagh 2009). In working with adults along the trauma continuum, what is important is not the availability of any verifiable truth, but the perception the client holds and makes the practitioner witness to (Clarkson 2009). Thus, although practitioners should always believe anything and everything a client discloses of his or her own accord, they should avoid cuing or colluding by viewing the client's story as a form of subjective, narrative truth, which may or may not be the same as objectively verifiable, historic truth of the sort required in law (Sabbagh 2009).

> In response to the client who asks "You do believe me don't you?," the safest response may be a variation of: "What you have just told me sounds dreadful, and I can see how disturbing it is when you retell it, or are reminded of it, and as your genetic counselor, I want to do the best I can to make this process as easy as possible for you. And I will need you to tell me how best to do this." The words, tone, and body language that the practitioner uses to communicate this will determine how empathically and congruently the message is transmitted and received.

Avoiding Boundary Breaches

As Courtois suggests:

> Clear role definition and boundary maintenance are especially relevant in the treatment of abuse survivors. Interpersonal victimization, by definition, involves the violation of personal boundaries. Chronic victimization further

involves conditioning into a relationship with overlapping roles, boundary slippage, ambivalent attachment, and ambivalent emotions. This affiliative conditioning may play out in other relationships including therapy. (1999: 161)

The work of all health professionals is boundaried by roles, rules, responsibilities, and relationships, described by Phillips et al. (2011) as the "4R's" of ethical boundary management that circumscribe the practitioner's remit and are prescribed by their employer, organization, regulatory bodies and in some cases the law. Despite this, the literature indicates that the members of all professions behave irrationally sometimes by breaching one or more of the "4R's" with or without negative consequences (Phillips 2006; Smith & Fitzpatrick 1995; Sutherland 2007). However, when working with the victims of sexual abuse, as a form of appropriate, compensatory, attachment, the working alliance and psychological contract depend on the maintenance of a consistent and securely boundaried relationship (Clarkson 2009; Green 2004; Rothschild 2000; Wilson & Keane 2004; Yule 2003). The more explicitly the "4R's" are articulated and adhered to, the less likely the practitioner is to fall prey to conflicts of interests and the occupational hazards and treatment traps outlined above. As the case study in Box 7.2 indicates, this will be influenced by a number of factors, such as the practitioner's limitations, his or her own agenda, personality, need for autonomy, or inability to tolerate the organizational constrictions that circumscribe the context of his or her practice.

The Case for Consultative Supervision

The experience of Susan's genetic counselor illustrates how even experienced practitioners can benefit from ongoing supervision (Clarke et al. 2007), the need for which increases for those working with traumatized clients (Clarkson 2009; Rothschild 2006). How confident and competent a practitioner is with the content, processes, and interactions involved in their work; their ability to disengage as well as engage appropriately with clients; and the extent to which they are willing to work within the parameters of the "4R's" are fundamental aspects of reflective practice in counseling supervision (Phillips et al. 2012). However, as Page (1999) observes "merely attending supervision does not necessarily result in any significant benefit to either client of counselor. It is the quality of work within the supervisory session that determines the effectiveness of outcome." Openness and honesty are essential components of effective supervision and reflective practice and, as this case illustrates, there is significant value in using a suitably qualified and experienced consultative supervisor from another discipline (Freeth 2007; Hansen, Himes, & Meier 1990; Morrissette 1996), one who, distinct from any hierarchical, managerial relationship, is able to help the practitioner consider the multiple perspectives to his or her practice (Hay 2007; Johns 2004). This form of supervision can provide the necessary conditions for the practitioner to reveal his or her fragilities and vulnerabilities more readily and help him or her to explore countertransference reactions—why he or she may get stuck, overinvolved, or out of his or her depth with certain clients (Sussman, 1995). Support and development is most effective when tailored to different specialities (Hackett & Palmer 2010), and, when provided by a suitably qualified and experienced supervisor who is able to perform the roles of educator, counselor, coach, and mentor, this can facilitate the normative, formative, and restorative components necessary to develop the practitioner's confidence and competence to practice with a range of clients (Proctor 2004). As an important parallel process (Hawkins & Shohet, 2005) designed to reinforce the supervisee's own internal supervisor (Casement 2004, 2008), the supervisor provides the necessary conditions for the promotion of a safe, open, and honest psychological contract and sound working alliance that serves as a model of good practice for the conditions necessary for working with the adult client who has been sexually abused as a child. In the case study in Box 7.2, by using an holistic, integrative and multi-modal approach that valued the counselor's feelings as well as thoughts and behaviors, in relation to the content, processes and interactions involved in genetic counseling the supervisor was able to proactively consider her unconscious, as well as conscious motivations, and, in this way rectify the dilemmas, occupational hazards, and treatment traps she had fallen foul of.

SUMMARY

The case studies presented here have only allowed a small glimpse into the insidious, enduring, and pervasive nature of childhood sexual abuse along a trauma continuum encompassing many permutations. However, in highlighting the complexity of working with adult survivors of this client population, they have allowed consideration of certain key implications and learning points for the genetic counselor and other health professionals. As childhood victims, these clients could not prevent the abuse of power perpetrated by adults who took advantage of their vulnerability. Therefore, as professionals, we need to be aware of the implications associated with the power imbalance inherent in the roles we perform in medical settings and the different ways in which the original trauma, associated with powerlessness, can be reenacted in this setting. As well as considering the needs of the client, much evidence exists to link practitioner health and well-being to the quality of client care (Beeston & Jeeson 1999; National Association for Staff Support and Royal College of Nursing [NASS:RCN] 1992; National Institute for Health and Clinical Excellence [NICE] 2009) and in considering certain dilemmas, occupational hazards, and treatment traps associated with this client population, we have seen how practitioners can prepare the environment and manage the content, processes, and interactions involved at each stage of the consultation to provide the optimum conditions for the health and well-being of client and practitioner alike. Practitioners in medical genetic and other health professions do not have to be trauma specialists to work with even deeply damaged survivors of abuse if they work safely and effectively by understanding the client's needs and their own ability to meet them. This includes the knowledge and self-awareness to explain what you can't as well as can offer; by being a reflective practitioner and knowing the limits of your confidence and competence to practice; and, when necessary, knowing how, when, and where to refer the client for specialist support prior to the particular stages and procedures of genetic counseling.

To this end, the following key learning points are suggested:

- For some clients, the abuse may not yet have surfaced fully. Practitioners will not know at what stage the client will be in recovery, and the experience of genetic counseling and family history-taking may trigger flashbacks.
- The possibility of abuse should be held in the practitioner's mind at all times and, because survivors of abuse are not readily identifiable, family histories should be taken with caution.
- Even for clients who are fully aware of their abuse and have had extensive therapy, there is always the possibility of further unexpected triggers, and inappropriate requests and responses can exacerbate the situation.
- Allow the client to talk and express his or her feelings however distressing this may be to the practitioner. It may be the first time the client has spoken of the issue, and it is vitally important that he or she is heard and believed.
- Ask the client what he or she needs and how you, as a genetic counselor, can support him or her. If a medical record cannot be made because of alienation by, or fear of relatives, discuss alternatives. And make it clear which family records are essential or only preferable.
- Do not assume that other relatives will provide support. Victims of abuse may have dysfunctional or nonexistent relationships with their family, and, if the predictive genetic test is positive, they may have no close support network.
- Do not assume that the abuser is male. For those assaulted by their mothers, female clinicians may be difficult to work with. Equally, do not assume that a male client will not have been abused by either parent or adults of both genders.
- The physical intrusiveness of tests may not be manageable, and injections and other routine blood tests can be highly problematic for people who have been sexually abused as it may represent a symbolic invasion—or reactivate memories of an actual invasion—of their body.
- Assume that medical processes will be difficult. Claustrophobia may be an issue (e.g. MRI scans), and colonoscopies or mammograms may be traumatizing. Ask clients which parts of any testing or medical process they are likely to find difficult and discuss alternatives or ways of managing it.
- In addition to the normal anxiety of waiting for a result, this can tip the abused person into trauma. Extra support or speeding up results should be offered, along with telephone consultations as an alternative to obligatory hospital site visits.

- Recognize potential phobias associated with medical settings and how a sense of powerlessness can tap into previous victimhood. As far as possible, remove clinical equipment, screens, and the like. Do not wear white coats, and ask other colleagues to remove theirs.

- Having to repeat the abuse history each time the client goes for a check-up and the need to explain why things need to be done differently will occur unless clinicians clearly record and highlight the abuse and the client's preferences in their records. For example, an explanation of why students cannot observe and why co-counseling should be avoided.

- When in doubt, the practitioner can avoid most treatment traps by going back to basics and asking themselves the following questions:

  - How confident and competent am I to work with the content, processes, and interactions required with this client?

  - How reasonable are the client's requests and my responses?

  - What is my role as a genetic counselor?

  - What rules apply to my role and this client group (policies, procedures, protocols, precedents, etc.)?

  - What are my responsibilities for, and to, this client as a genetic counselor?

  - What is my professional relationship to this client?

REFERENCES

American Psychiatric Association. (1994). *Diagnostic and Statistical Manual of Mental Disorders* (4th ed.). Washington, DC: Author.

Beeston, H., & Jeeston, A. (1999). Caring for staff: Setting quality standards. *Nursing Standard, 13*(36), 43–45.

Berne, E. (1968). *Games people play*. London: Penguin Books.

Brewin, C. R. (2003). *Post-traumatic stress disorder: Malady or myth?* London: Yale University Press

Casement, P. (2004). *On learning from the patient*. London: Routledge.

Casement, P. (2008). *Learning from our mistakes: Beyond dogma in psychoanalysis and psychotherapy*. London: Routledge.

Clarke, A., Middleton, A., Cowley, L., Guilbert, P., Macleod, R., & Tran, V. (2007). Report from the UK and Eire Association of Genetic Nurses and Counsellors (AGNC) supervision working group on genetic counselling supervision. *Journal of Genetic Counselling, 6*(2), 127–142.

Clarkson, P. (2009). *The therapeutic relationship*. London: Whurr Publishers.

Courtois, C. A. (1999). *Recollections of sexual abuse: Treatment principles and guidelines*. New York: Norton.

Cozolino, L. (2002). *The neuroscience of psychotherapy*. New York: Norton.

Evans, C. (2006). *Genetic counselling: A psychological approach*. Cambridge, UK: Cambridge Press.

Frederickson, R. (1992). *Repressed memories: A journey to recovery from sexual abuse*. New York: Simon & Schuster.

Freeth, R. (2007). *Humanising psychiatry and mental health care: The challenge of the person-centred approach*. Oxford, UK: Radcliffe Publishing.

Gilbert, P. (2009). *The compassionate mind*. London: Constable & Robinson.

Green, V. (2004). *Emotional development in psychoanalysis, attachment theory and neuroscience: Creating connections*. New York: Brunner-Routledge.

Hackett, A., & Palmer, S. (2010). An investigation into the perceived stressors for staff working in the hospice service. *International Journal of Palliative Nursing, 16*(6), 290–296.

Hansen, J., Himes, B., & Meier, S. (1990). *Consultation: Concepts and practices*. Englewood Cliffs, NJ: Prentice-Hall.

Hawkins, P., & Shohet, R. (2005). *Supervision in the helping professions*. Maidenhead, UK: Open University Press.

Hay, J. (2007). *Reflective practice and supervision for coaches*. Maidenhead, UK: Open University Press.

Johns, C. (2004). *Becoming a reflective practitioner* (2nd ed.). Oxford, UK: Blackwell Publishing.

Karpman, S. B. (1968). Fairy tales and script drama analysis. *Transactional Analysis Bulletin, 17*(26).

Kinchin, D. (2005). *Post traumatic stress disorder: The invisible injury*. Didcot, UK: Success Unlimited.

Kreger, R. (2008). *The essential family guide to borderline personality disorder*. Center City, MN: Hazelden Information Services.

Malone, C. (1996). *The memory birds: Survivors of sexual abuse*. London: Virago.

McCann, L., & Pearlman, L. A. (1990). Vicarious traumatisation: A framework for understanding the psychological effects of working with victims. *Journal of Traumatic Stress, 3*, 131–149.

McNally, R. J. (2003). *Remembering trauma*. London: Belknap Harvard University Press.

Morrissette, P. J. (1996). Family therapist as consultant in foster care: Expanding the parameters of practice. *American Journal of Family Therapy, 24*, 55–64.

National Association for Staff Support and Royal College of Nursing (NASS:RCN). (1992). *Charter for staff support*. London: RCN.

National Institute for Health and Clinical Excellence (NICE). (2009). *Promoting mental wellbeing through productive and healthy working conditions: Guidance for employers*. Accessed March 3, 2012 from http://www.nice.org.uk/nicemedia/pdf/PH22Guidance.pdf

Page, S. (1999). *The shadow and the counsellor: Working with darker aspects of the person, role and profession*. New York: Routledge.

Phillips, A. (2006). Light out of darkness: Alder Hey assessed. *Healthcare Counselling and Psychotherapy Journal, 24*(3), 22–25.

Phillips, A., Mannion, G., & Birch. J. (2012). Crafting practice: Through consultatice supervision. *Healthcare Counselling and Psychotherapy Journal, 12*(2), 30–33.

Proctor, B. (2004). *Group supervision: A guide to creative practice*. London: Sage.

Rothschild, B. (2000). *The body remembers: The psychophysiology of trauma and trauma treatment*. New York: Norton.

Rothschild, B. (2006). *Help for the helper: The psychophysiology of compassion fatigue and vicarious trauma*. New York: Norton.

Sabbagh, K. (2009). *Remembering childhood trauma: How memory betrays us*. Oxford, UK: Oxford University Press.

Scott, M. J. (2008). *Moving on after trauma*. Hove, UK: Routledge.

Smith, D., & Fitzpatrick, M. (1995). Patient-therapist boundary issues: An integrative review of theory and research. *Professional Psychology: Research and Practice, 26*(50), 499–506.

Spinelli, E. (2009). *Demystifying therapy*. Ross-on-Wye, UK: PCCS Books.

Sussman, M. B. (1995). *A perilous calling: The hazards of psychotherapy practice*. New York: John Wiley & Sons Inc.

Sutherland, S. (2007). *Irrationality*. London: Pinter & Martin.

Wilson, J. P., & Keane, T. M. (eds.). (2004). *Assessing psychological trauma and PTSD*. New York: Guildford Press.

Wilson, J. P., & Lindy, J. D. (1994). *Counter transference in the treatment of PTSD*. New York: Guilford Press.

Yule, W. (2003). *Post-traumatic stress disorders: Concepts and therapy*. Chichester, UK: Wiley & Sons.

8 Communicating with Teenagers

Anna Gregorowski

The dead might as well try to speak to the living as the old to the young.
—Willa Cather

Communicating effectively with adolescents requires both an interest in working with young people and a set of skills that can be learned along the way. Many health professionals do not like communicating with young people, as the stereotypical view is one of uncommunicative individuals unwilling to engage with adults. Health professionals can also feel ill equipped to work with adolescents, especially when there is little understanding of adolescent lifestyle issues due to a lack of training in this area. Although working with this age group may present some challenges for the health professional, it also presents opportunities for engagement and health promotion. Communicating with adolescents can be exciting and rewarding if the health professional is keen to learn the skills for effective communication with this age group and has the support to do this.

Adolescence is a time of vast change, when physical, mental, and social development occur at a rapid rate, with biological development occurring faster than at any time other than during prenatal life (Waddell 1998). Adolescents have different health needs to those of children and adults, needs that change as physical development and accompanying psychosocial changes occur. It is also a time when future health behaviors and outcomes are determined (Viner 2005).

Growing evidence suggests that the adolescent brain is different from both the child's and the adult's brain (Steinberg 2010). These differences translate into increased vulnerability in adolescents through increased risk-taking behavior.

> **Box 8.1** HEEADSSS
>
> H   Home life, including relationships with parents and siblings
>
> E   Education or employment
>
> E   Eating
>
> A   Activities (peer related) including sport
>
> D   Drugs including alcohol and cigarette use
>
> S   Sexual history/relationships
>
> S   Suicidality, self-harm, and depression
>
> S   Safety

If communication is to be effective, it is crucial that health professionals respond appropriately to young people. They can use the opportunity for developing rapport, positive role modeling, and health promotion. This chapter aims to help health professionals to communicate effectively with adolescents. It outlines why young people should be treated differently from children and adults, and is written at a time when adolescent medicine is emerging as a discipline in its own right. Adolescent health incorporates a communication framework (HEEADSSS, see Box 8.1) that can be adapted for clinical practice. The chapter sets out top tips on communication with young people in all settings, using a case study to illustrate the principles of getting it "good enough" for effective communication to take place.

BACKGROUND

The numbers of adolescents aged 10 to 19 years living in the United Kingdom has increased from 7.0 million in 1995 to 7.6 million in 2009, with slightly more adolescents than children under 10 years (7.2 million) at present (Coleman et al. 2011).

It is useful to start by considering various definitions of adolescence. The World Health Organization defines adolescence as the second decade of life (10–20 years) and defines "youth" as being from 10 to 25 years of age. Although adolescence can be referred to as the period between childhood and adulthood, finding a useful working definition of adolescence can be challenging. It is more useful to think about adolescence using a biopsychosocial model rather than using a chronological definition (Viner 2005). Physically, adolescence is about biological maturation. It starts with the onset of puberty and ends with growth completion. This is a variable process between boys and girls, can be affected by chronic illness, and is variable between individuals as each develops at his or her own rate. Psychosocially, it is about becoming more independent. This is achieved through developing an identity, seeking out a peer group, functioning more autonomously in terms of travel and socializing, and developing more adult ways of thinking.

PREPARING FOR THE CONSULTATION

It is useful to start consultation preparation by thinking through the possible biopsychosocial development of the client. This can be done by considering who referred the young person. Who is anxious that they are seen? What is the expectation that information will be fed back? How will this be managed? If possible, send preappointment information about the consultation to the client: who the young person will see, the length of appointment, what to bring, and that there will be an opportunity to be seen privately. It is useful to include the expectation that seeing the young person privately is usual (normalizing model).

If possible, try to offer "adolescent" or "transition" clinics as seeing similarly aged young people in the same clinic is helpful. If numbers of clients in this age group are not sufficient, group clients of a similar age at the beginning or end of the clinic. This is good for peer support and allows for the environment to be laid out and information provided appropriately for young people. If possible, provide adolescent clinics after school or at weekends. This helps to minimize disruption for young people who are at school, in college, or working. It is good practice to offer written and, if possible, web-based information that is age appropriate and ideally available in different languages. This information should describe the service and provide sign-posting to other relevant services (mental health, sexual health), before and after the appointment.

COMMUNICATION IN THE CONSULTATION

Adolescence is a time of rapid physical change, with accompanying shifts in psychological development and social function. Using a communication framework that is holistic and flexible in approach is sensible. The HEEADSSS tool (Box 8.1) does this and is widely accepted among experts in adolescent health throughout the world.

HEEADSSS provides an opportunity to develop rapport with a young person, guides intervention, and encompasses risk assessment. It is best used when the adolescent is relatively well, but can be adapted and used in smaller sections when the adolescent is not well or in crisis. It is designed to be used in a 20-minute consultation, but can take longer to complete if the adolescent is in distress or a topic is explored in more depth.

Before starting on the HEEADSSS assessment, be sure to explain confidentiality: "What we talk about together will remain private, unless it is in your or another person's best interest to share information you have shared. I will let you know if I feel it is important to share anything that we talk about today with someone else. I will explain who I will share it with and why, and I'll discuss with you how I might do that."

By assuring confidentiality in any communication with a young person, including explaining what this means and when you might need to talk to another professional or a parent about a concerning issue that the young person communicates to you, you let the young person know that it is fine to share as much, or as little, as he or she wishes to communicate. Be clear about follow-up and future communication. If the young person knows that there is another opportunity for communication or that this is an ongoing process, he or she may choose to share information at a different pace.

> Try to see young people by themselves, as well as with their parents. There are many things that young people may not discuss with a parent present—like relationship issues, sexual health, and drug or alcohol use. Conversely, there are other issues that they may want their parent to be present for—medication and treatment changes are two examples of times when adolescents often prefer a parent to be present. Offering opportunities for young people to be seen alone, or with a family member or a peer present, gives the young person a choice and some control over how communication happens.

After explaining confidentiality, you can then begin the consultation with "problem free" talk. This provides an opportunity to assess protective factors from the start. Explain how the consultation is likely to be structured: how long it will last; that it contains a number of routine topics that will help you to understand more about the young person—his or her strengths and what he or she finds challenging, where he or she lives, who his or her friends are, and how he or she likes to spend time; what has changed because he or she is not well. Emphasize confidentiality from the outset and encourage the young person to ask questions along the way.

Start with general questions then become more specific. If the young person answers yes to a question, ask more, and, if not, move on to the next question. Before some questions, you can normalize the content "some young people tell us that they feel so low that they want to hurt themselves, have you ever felt like that?" Even if you are really worried about a young person, share your concerns with them in a calm way and, if you do decide to break confidentiality, explain your rationale for doing so and agree to a plan of next steps with the young person

HEEADSSS TECHNIQUE

HEEADSSS provides a range of questions centring around:

Home: Asking about a young person's home life is usually a neutral place to start.

Education/Employment: Asking about this can give you an idea of how a young person is spending his or her time and also of how he or she is doing in terms of academic or financial progress.

Eating: This section has been more recently added and contains useful questions about eating habits and mealtimes. It also gives an insight into a young person's shape or weight concerns if they have any.

Activities: Ask about what type of activities, including sports, a young person is engaged in. This gives an idea about what interests him or her and whether he or she prefers to do things alone, with friends, or with family members, and also whether he or she is sports-minded or prefers other types of activities.

Drug use: This includes cigarettes and alcohol, and other drug usage can provide insight and an opportunity for health promotion as appropriate.

Sex: This includes asking about relationships and provides an opportunity to talk about contraception.

Suicide: This starts with talking about mood and is an important part of communication with a young person—it should include asking about self-harm and suicide, whenever you are concerned about the way a young person is presenting or about what he or she is telling you.

Safety: This has also been recently added and explores with the young person how safe he or she is in his or her everyday lives and whether there are any safety factors that may impinge on his or her general health and well-being.

A Note on Assessing Risk

Many health professionals are not used to assessing risk and have had little or no training in this area. It is important, even with little formal training in this, to be able to do a basic strengths and risk assessment as part of any adolescent consultation. During the consultation, remember to ask—don't assume! In any communication with a young person, a good place to begin is by asking what the young person hopes to gain from the interaction. Do they want to be seen in the clinic? What hopes— and fears—do they bring to the communication? What information do they hope to leave with? Do they want to be seen alone or with a friend or parent?

Here are a few guidelines to consider when assessing strengths and risk:

- *Consider strengths and risk alongside each other.* The flip side of risk in a young person's life are the protective factors, and thinking with the young person about the balance between the two is helpful. For example, if a young person is feeling low in mood (risk) but talks to a parent or friend when feeling this way (protective factor), there is less concern than if the young person withdraws or isolates him- or herself (risk) when feeling low.
- *Start with general questions then become more specific.* If the young person answers yes to a question, ask more—if not, move onto the next question
- *Before some questions, normalize the content.* For example: "Some young people tell us that they feel so low that they want to hurt themselves, have you ever felt like that?"

- *It can be useful to ask a young person to score his or her mood.* Use a scale of 1–10 (where 1 is the lowest in mood and 10 the highest). Ask for an average score for the past week and what his or her highest and lowest in the past week has been. This can generate discussion (i.e., "When you are feeling 8 out of 10, what is happening for you? What about when you are more like 2 out of 10? What is happening for you? Do you talk to anyone about how you are feeling? Do you think about self-harm? Do you follow this through?")
- *Share your concerns in a calm way.* If you do decide to break confidentiality, explain your rationale for doing so and agree to a plan of next steps with the young person.

Toward the end of the consultation, discuss with the young person what he or she is happy to share with parents (especially if the parents are joining for the latter part of the appointment). Also discuss what will be recorded in the clinical notes, clinic letters, or reports. Recording a summary of topics discussed without too much detail can be useful if the young person is keen to keep the details of the consultation private. End the interview with problem-free talk.

Be yourself. One thing that young people tell us is that they do not like to speak to adults who try to be cool or pretend to be what they are not. Being yourself includes being honest when you do not know the answer to a question. It is better to let a young person know that you do not have all the answers, but are willing to either find or signpost them to some answers. Signposting adolescents to sources of information can help to empower the young person and help him or her to find his or her own answers, which helps to improve his or her confidence.

Use appropriate language—think about the age and stage of development of the young person you are communicating with, and try to use language that is as age appropriate as possible. Find out what the young person already knows and ask what he or she is hoping to gain through the communication. This can help the interaction get off to a good start (see Box 8.2).

Box 8.2 Case Study

Kate is a 16-year-old girl with cystic fibrosis and diabetes mellitus. She has not been adhering to medication/treatment for the past 2 years, and has twice been hospitalized with chest infections and once with diabetic ketoacidosis (DKA) in the past year. She recently started junior college, where she met her boyfriend, Jake. Jake is 17 years old. Kate has been told about cystic fibrosis and how it is an inherited condition, but she is not sure of all the facts and feels embarrassed to ask. She is worried that Jake will want to have sex with her. She has not been sexually active before and is not sure what contraceptive method to use.

(continued)

Box 8.2 (continued)

Kate currently lives at home with her mom, stepdad, her brother Sam, who is 13 years old and well, and two younger stepsiblings, aged 8 and 6. She and her mother argue a lot (about medication/treatment, school, Kate's boyfriend, and Kate's eating habits). Kate is keen to leave home soon but does not have money. She has two girlfriends whom she is close to, but one of them does not like Jake. She does not smoke but does drink (wine or spirits) at parties.

She has tried to get more information about her illness and contraception on the Internet, but is increasingly confused with the information that she has found. She is not keen to come to see you as her mom arranged the appointment. She decides to come and see you anyway, as she feels desperate.

In preparing to see Kate, consider: who referred Kate, what information you might be expected to share with Kate's mother and how you will manage this, how you will provide a quiet and private environment for the consultation, how to communicate with Kate and her mother before you see her, and that it is your usual practice to see young people on their own for confidential consultations.

Explaining confidentiality and what the consultation would include helped Kate to feel more in control of her situation. When the professional discussed with Kate that they could agree what to feed back to her mother, Kate felt she was being given a choice, which helped to further increase her sense of being in control and enabled her to talk more freely. The HEEADSSS framework gave a direction of travel to the time spent together and for exploring topics in a safe way. Kate responded well to this, letting the professional know what she would like to explore further and also what she would not like to talk about at that time. Together, Kate and the professional identified that Kate would find it helpful to know more about her illnesses and the effect of growing up, and about the impact of lifestyle choices on her health. The professional signposted her to the relevant clinical nurse specialist (CNS) and provided written contact details for this professional. They also discussed sexual health and relationship issues. This provided Kate with a space to think about whether she felt ready for a physical relationship with her new boyfriend and also what contraception she might use. She was also signposted to a sexual health service for more information.

The professional undertook a mini risk assessment on Kate (her lowest, highest, and average mood scored between 1 and 10 for the past week, where 10 is the happiest). Kate scored herself at 4/10 (when worrying about her illness, or feeling under pressure from her mother or boyfriend), 8/10 (out shopping with girlfriends, or at a movie), and 7/10 (most of the time). No risk concerns were identified.

Toward the end of the consultation, Kate agreed to another meeting with the professional in a week's time. Kate left feeling listened to and with a plan in mind to address some of the knowledge gaps with the CNS's help. She agreed to let her mother know that she would be seeing the professional again in a week's time as she and the professional thought this would be reassuring to her mother and stop her asking questions or pressuring Kate further.

SUMMARY

Here are some tips for more effective communication with young people.

- Be clear about what you want to assess before you begin.
- Making a good beginning can affect the whole consultation—take time to explain what the consultation is about and answer questions.
- Be honestly interested in what the young person has to say; taking a curious, nonintrusive, and respectful stance can be helpful.
- Progress from neutral to more sensitive topics.
- Don't rush. Take your time, especially at the beginning or when exploring sensitive issues.
- Check that the young person has understood what you are saying at regular intervals, without appearing condescending.
- Be flexible; tailor what you do and how you do it to the situation.
- Use language that is clear, age-appropriate, and easily understood, and interactive rather than interrogative.
- Listen carefully to answers and to what is left unsaid, being aware of body language—yours and the young person's—in the consultation.
- Take "third-person" approach.
- Respect the adolescent's concerns and points of view.
- Respect confidentiality.
- Negotiate what to feed back.

Useful HEEADSSS questions (adapted from Goldenring & Rosen 2004) include:

H: Where do you live? Who lives with you? How do you get along with your family? Who could you talk to if you needed help with a problem? What do your mom and dad do? Have you moved recently? Ever run away? Is there anyone new at home?

E: What do you like/not like about school/work? What can you do well/what areas would you like to improve on? How do you get along with teachers/ other students? How well do you do at school? Has this changed recently? Have you ever been suspended from school? Many young people experience bullying at school—have you ever been bullied?

E: Sometimes when people are stressed, they can overeat or undereat. Have you ever experienced either of these? In general, what is your diet like? Do you ever restrict your eating? Are you happy with your weight and the way you look?

A: What do you like to do with friends? What do you do for fun? Where? When? What do you do with family? Do you play sport? What hobbies do you do? Tell me about the parties you go to. How much TV do you watch each day/night? Do you use the computer every day? Facebook? Xbox? Play Station? What games do you like to play? Favorite music? Have you ever been in trouble for breaking the law?

D: Many people at your age are starting to experiment with cigarettes and/or alcohol. Have any of your friends tried these or maybe other drugs like marijuana, IV drugs, etc.? How about you, have you tried any? Ask about the effects of drug-taking/smoking or alcohol on them, and any regrets. How much are they taking, how often, and has frequency increased recently?

S: Some people are getting involved in sexual relationships. Have you had a sexual experience with a guy or girl or both? Are you comfortable with these experiences? Did you use contraception? If yes, what type? Has anyone ever touched you in a way that's made you feel uncomfortable or forced you into a sexual relationship? (History of sexual or physical abuse.) How do you feel about relationships in general/about your own sexuality?

S: How do you feel in yourself at the moment on a scale of 1–10? What sort of things do you do if you are feeling sad, angry, or hurt? Is there anyone you can talk to? Do you feel this way often? Some people who feel really down often feel like hurting themselves or even killing themselves. Have you ever felt this way? Have you ever tried to hurt yourself or take your own life? What have you tried? What prevented you from doing so? Do you feel the same way now? Have you made a plan?

S: Ask about use of sun protection, immunization, bullying, carrying weapons, coping techniques such as their beliefs, religion, music, what helps them to relax.

FURTHER READING

Department of Health. (2004). *National service framework for children, young people and maternity services*. London: Author.

Department of Health. (2006). *Transition: Getting it right for young people*. Publication Code 271558/Transition: Getting it right for young people. London: Author.

Department of Health. (2008). *Transition: Moving on well* Publication Code 284732/ Transition: Moving on well. London: Author.

Department of Health. (2010). *You're welcome*. Available at www.dh.gov.uk/en/ PublicationsAndStatistics/Publications/PublicationsPolicyAndGuidance/DH_4121562

Department of Health. (2010). *You're welcome quality assessment toolkit*. Available at www. dh.gov.uk/en/Publicationsandstatistics/Publications/PublicationsPolicyAndGuidance/ DH_097571

General Medical Council. (2007). *0–18 years guidance: Communication*. London: .

General Medical Council. (2008). *Consent: Patients and doctors making decisions together*. London.

General Medical Council. (2009). *Confidentiality*. London

Royal College of General Practice. (2011). *Confidentiality and young people: Improving teenagers uptake of sexual and other health advice*. Available from www.rcgp.org.uk ISBN 0-85084-269-7

REFERENCES

Coleman, J., Brooks, F., & Treadgold, P. (2011). *Key data on adolescence 2011* London: Association for Young People's Health.

Goldenring, J., & Rosen, D. (2004). Getting into adolescent heads: An essential update. *Contemporary Pediatrics, 21*(1):64–90.

Steinberg, L. (2010). A behavioural scientist looks at the science of adolescent brain development. *Brain and Cognition, 72,*160–164.

Viner, R. (2005). *ABC of adolescence* (pp. 1–4). London: Wiley-Blackwell.

Waddell, M. (1998). *Inside lives: Psychoanalysis and the growth of the personality (pp. 125–155)*. London: Duckworth.

9 Communicating with Children Who Have Intellectual Disability

Jeremy Turk

We worry about what a child will become tomorrow, yet we forget that he is someone today.

—Stacia Tauscher

Psychological difficulties in childhood and adolescence can comprise emotional, behavioral, temperamental, and developmental problems (Turk, Graham, & Verhulst 2007). These are all now acknowledged as having substantial genetic predispositions, which are then influenced by psychological and social aspects and experiences (McGuffin & Rutter 2002).

Developmental difficulties are particularly prevalent and are usually of early onset, long term, and frequently multiple. In addition to intellectual disability, individuals often experience social, communicatory, and obsessional tendencies consistent with autism spectrum conditions (ASC) (Wing 2003), and inattentiveness, restlessness, fidgetiness, impulsiveness, and distractibility consistent with attention deficit-hyperactivity disorder (ADHD) (Merwood & Asherson 2011).

Emotional and behavioral difficulties in childhood can often be understood in terms of the individual's level of developmental functioning or mental age. They can also be understandable responses to experiences (life events, daily hassles) and the result of increased vulnerability due to associated intellectual disability. However, they can also be part of a general genetic predisposition to psychological problems (Turk 2007a), as well as being more specific to particular genetic disorders—so-called behavioral phenotypes (Turk 2007b). Indeed, temperamental tendencies within the general population are now known to have substantial genetic contributions (Plomin 2008).

With advances in human genome research, increasing numbers of genetic disorders are being confirmed as associated with intellectual disability, ASCs, and ADHD. Severe self-injurious tendencies also have a strong genetic basis, particularly in fragile X syndrome (Turk 2011), Lesch-Nyhan syndrome (Hall, Oliver, & Murphy 2001; Robey, Reck, Giacomini, Barabas, & Eddey 2003), Cornelia de Lange syndrome (Berney, Ireland, & Burn 1999; Oliver, Sloneem, Hall, & Arron 2009), Prader-Willi syndrome (Swillen, Verhoeven, & Fryns 2002), and Smith-Magenis syndrome (Shelley & Robertson 2005). Nonetheless, beneficial treatments are usually psychologically based (Oliver & Richards 2010; Turk 2004; Turk & O'Brien 2002) although judicious use of certain medications may ameliorate a number of challenging behaviors (Matson & Neale 2009).

Parents will often show some of their children's genetically determined psychological traits. For example, research confirms that first-degree relatives of autistic individuals have elevated rates of social and communicatory dysfunction, as well as heightened psychological rigidity, aloofness, anxiety, and hypersensitivity to criticism. (Piven et al. 1997)

These tendencies complicate other autistic features, which will often be present in the child, including literal thinking, social one-sidedness, lack of empathy and understanding, problems with the meaning and use of language, obsessional preoccupations and behaviors, and lack of imaginary play and skills. Parents of children with ADHD are said to have a one in three chance of displaying traits of the condition.

Information relating to the above is best provided to families in brief, clear, and concrete bites, with the counselor being mindful of short concentration spans, as well as parental exhaustion, anguish, distress, grief, and often a profound sense of guilt. Time needs to be provided for information to be absorbed and considered, and polite repetition as well as clear, concise, and simple written material is useful. Sharing information on support groups with individuals and their families is vital,

---

Box 9.1 Case Study

Andy, who is currently 10 years old, came to the attention of local child and adolescent mental health services 2 years previously following intensive social services involvement regarding severe psychosocial adversities. These included chronic neglect throughout his life as a result of his father's drug and alcohol problems. His mother had, under duress, colluded with his father in funding his drug habit through her children's state benefit. Andy and his brothers and sisters had also witnessed their father's verbal abuse of their mother. The father no longer lives with them. According to the social work report, the father had required compulsory psychiatric admission twice, and, on the second admission, was given a diagnosis of a drug-induced psychosis.

(continued)

Box 9.1 (continued)

On presentation to child and adolescent mental health services, Andy was quite incoherent and disoriented. He claimed to be hearing voices, seeing ghosts, and to be communicating regularly with a seagull that was following him. He also reported having nightmares, anxiety, and difficulty in sleeping. However, when interviewed by specialist child and adolescent mental health staff, he was calm and cooperative and played happily with a toy train set throughout the consultation. He seemed oriented in time, place, and person, and appeared to understand and give coherent answers to questions. Educational data confirmed longstanding struggling with school work, yielding an IQ in the mild intellectual disability range, which had been attributed to his social situation. Andy was also described educationally as having enormous difficulty concentrating, being quite restless and fidgety in class, and displaying markedly impulsive behaviors with high levels of distractibility. In addition, he was reported as finding social interaction and communicating with other children, including playing with them, difficult. As part of a general medical assessment, Andy's chromosomes were analyzed. This revealed Klinefelter syndrome. A decision was made to meet with Andy's mother in the first instance to share this information and its implications. The meeting was planned to occur in a comfortable room, within the local Child Development Center, with as few "trappings" of clinical practice as possible. The timing of the meeting was arranged to fit in as far as possible with the mother's childcare needs and arrangements. Those present sat on informal chairs round a low, small table. Efforts were made to ensure lack of interruptions and to minimize extraneous noise and other possible distractions. The recent positive good news of the family having been granted a ground floor apartment in a congenial and well-maintained local supported housing development was shared. So, too, was Andy's recent commencement on anticonvulsant medication for epilepsy. Mother described Andy's ambition to join the army, and his continuing morbid attraction to drug addicts and alcoholics. She also described his continuing high levels of emotional sensitivity, anxiety, and social passivity, in association with good levels of empathy and considerateness for others, and good behavior. Language and communication were continuing to be major areas of need, and concentration span was reported as still limited. Andy was continuing to receive regular psychological counseling at school.

Andy's mother was informed of the chromosome results and its nature, and implications were shared, along with plain-English written information and details of the national support group. It was agreed to meet again, this time with Andy present, to explore with him the diagnosis of Klinefelter syndrome and its implications. On this subsequent occasion, following a welcoming discussion with Andy as to the nature of the clinic and sharing about how he was getting on at home and school, a clear and simple explanation was given to him regarding his having Klinefelter syndrome. He was told that this makes him quite a special person—just like only 1 in 500 or so other people—in having a bit more of a special chemical called chromosomes than

(continued)

the rest of us. The doctor explained to him how most of us have 46 chromosomes, but he is special because he has 47. Andy was told how this was found out by the clever scientists looking at a bit of the blood that came out of his arm, by their looking down a microscope. It was explained to him that what this means is that we know a bit more about why he finds learning difficult and why he finds it difficult to behave himself and to get on with others sometimes. Recent achievements (Andy was very proud of becoming a seconder in the red six at Cubs and having a swimming badge) were applauded, and Andy shared how he was looking forward to Cub camp so he could get a camping badge as well, prior to graduating to Scouts and then hopefully fulfilling his ambition to join the army "because they have guns." Andy seemed very happy to be "special" and had no particular questions to ask about his diagnosis. He seemed relieved to know that his learning difficulties and his behavior problems were not entirely his fault. It was agreed that Andy should continue his supportive psycho-therapy and counseling, including work on his posttraumatic difficulties, and that his mother would be supported in her efforts to further stabilize the family social situation. Agreement was reached to reconvene at a later date to discuss any issues arising out of the shared information.

as is considering the use of pictorial in addition to written information and materials (see Box 9.1).

BACKGROUND

Developmental disabilities can be defined as early-onset, long-term, and frequently multiple psychological impairments that interfere with the normally fluent and spontaneous process of human skill acquisition, these skills being necessary for maximization of individual potential and quality of life (Turk 1996). These impairments produce adverse functional physical and psychological consequences, which, in turn, predispose to multiple and often severe social adversities and social disadvantage.

Developmental disabilities are usually subclassified into global and specific developmental disorders, also known as global and specific learning difficulties. The terms "global intellectual disability," "global developmental delay," "learning disability" and, in the United States, "mental retardation" are all used to describe global, early-onset, and long-term delays in skill acquisition so that the child's IQ should be less than approximately 70 and the child should be functionally impaired in everyday life skills. Two to three percent of children and young people qualify for such a term. Numerous synonyms have been used over time in efforts to counteract stigma associated with intellectual impairment. Redundant categories such as imbecile, idiot, and feeble-minded were initially replaced with concepts of mental or educational subnormality. Mental retardation is still the preferred term in North American clinical practice, where "learning disabilities" or "learning difficulties" refer more to specific developmental delays such as reading and spelling difficulties (dyslexia) and numeracy difficulties (dyscalculia). However, preschool-aged children are still often referred to as having "generalized developmental delay." Educationally, special schools and other educational services exist for children with "moderate" and "severe" learning difficulties, equivalent to IQ ranges of approximately 50–70 and less than 50, respectively.

Diagnostic and classificatory systems differ to some degree, and, as educational terminology is also different and some older terms persist, it is not surprising that confusion commonly occurs. Mild learning (or intellectual) disability differs from more severe forms in presentation, etiology, associated features, prevalence, appropriate management, and outcome. The distinction between the two on the basis of severity is therefore vital. Healthwise, intellectual or learning, disability is subclassified into mild (IQ 50–70), moderate (IQ 35–50), severe (IQ 20–35), and profound (IQ less than 25). Educationally, the term "learning difficulties" is preferred, and is divided into moderate learning difficulties (IQ 50–70), and severe learning difficulties (IQ less than 50).

These categories refer to delays, distortions, and disabilities relating to intellectual functioning or "cognition." However, two other important spectra of psychological developmental disabilities exist, both with major genetic underpinnings and implications.

The ASCs consist of multiple, qualitative, early-onset, and enduring impairments in a classic triad of psychological abilities (namely, social functioning, language, and communication and ritualistic and obsessional tendencies) (Wing 2003). Affected individuals also frequently experience multiple sensory sensitivities (Leekam, Nieto, Libby, Wing, & Gould 2007), impairments in imaginative and symbolic skills, and gross and fine motor difficulties. Recent estimates suggest that as many as 1%–2% of the population have an ASC (Baron-Cohen et al. 2009). However, only approximately 5% have an IQ above average, and 70% also experience intellectual disability. There is overwhelming evidence for a highly genetic basis in most instances of ASC (Kumar & Christian 2009). This evidence derives from twin, sibling, family, and adoption studies. Parents of individuals with ASC have also been found to have higher than expected rates and levels of associated features, notably psychological rigidity, social aloofness, hypersensitivity to criticism, and high anxiety levels (Piven et al. 1997). Families also frequently contain individuals with related developmental difficulties covering social, communicatory, and cognitive anomalies (Losh et al. 2009).

The ADHDs consist of similarly early-onset and enduring multiple developmental disabilities, in this instance affecting concentration ability and attentiveness, restlessness, fidgetiness, impulsiveness, distractibility, and mental organization ("executive function") skills (Banaschewski, Coghill Danckaerts, & Döpfner 2009). There may or may not be associated chaotic and disorganized gross motor overactivity. Prevalence rates suggest that 3%–5% of individuals may qualify for having an ADHD (Polanczyk, de Lima, Horta, Biederman, & Rohde 2007). North American nomenclature, being adopted increasingly in Europe and elsewhere, describes three subtypes, ADHD predominantly overactive and impulsive type, ADHD predominantly inattentive type, and ADHD combined type. The last, the most serious, affects 0.5%–1% of individuals, reportedly boys more than girls, and is synonymous with the European term "hyperkinetic disorder." Frequently, multiple features of intellectual disability, ASCs, and ADHD coexist in the same individual, thus increasing the complexity of assessment and treatment, and reflecting the need to label all areas of developmental disability for any one person rather than reducing his or her diagnosis to a single word or phrase.

There also exist an array of specific developmental disabilities that represent difficulties in particular psychological functions. These include

- *Dyslexia*: Language and spelling difficulties
- *Dyscalculia*: Numeracy difficulties
- *Dysphasia*: Word finding difficulties
- *Dysarthria*: Coordination of language production difficulties
- *Dyspraxia*: Fine motor coordination difficulties
- *Sensory hypersensitivities* or overfascinations with sight, sound, taste, touch, smell

Mental Health and Psychiatric Disorder in Young People

Approximately 7% of children and young people have a diagnosable psychiatric disorder. The rate increases to approximately 11% in those who experience the psychological adversities of having a chronic physical condition such as congenital heart disease, inflammatory bowel disease, or childhood-onset diabetes. The presence of central nervous system anomalies, as in epilepsy (Buelow et al. 2003) and cerebral palsy (Parkes et al. 2008), increases the rate further to approximately 33%. Children and young people with moderate to profound intellectual disability have a 50% rate of mental disorder. All these rates can be doubled when the predisposing factors coexist with significant degrees of social disadvantage, deprivation, adversity, abuse, or neglect. Hence, in any child with developmental disability and/or a mental health problem, it is important to clarify whether the associated emotional and behavioral difficulties and challenges are:

- consistent with the individual's general level of developmental functioning or "mental age"
- understandable responses to experiences and life events
- contributed to by the vulnerability of having intellectual disability
- indicative of a specific developmental delay
- part of a general genetic predisposition to psychopathology
- part of the characteristic profile of psychological and developmental difficulties associated with a specific genetic condition ("behavioral phenotype").

Autism

Research confirms that autism can be a presenting feature of a number of genetic conditions, for example fragile X syndrome (Turk & Graham 1997), untreated phenylketonuria (Baieli, Pavone, Meli, Fiumara, & Coleman 2003), neurofibromatosis (Johnson, Wiggs, Stores, & Huson 2005), tuberous sclerosis (Curatolo, Napolioni, & Moavero 2010), and Cohen syndrome (Howlin, Karpf, & Turk 2005).

It is now possible to make associations between specific profiles of autistic social and communicatory challenges and particular underlying genetic anomalies. Individuals with fragile X syndrome tend to be friendly and sociable, albeit somewhat shy and socially anxious, with repetitive and echoed speech. Tuberous sclerosis is often associated with marked stubbornness, oppositionalism, and defiance, along with overactivity and inattentiveness. Angelman syndrome is associated with high rates of social aloofness and social passivity. Individuals with Turner syndrome are characteristically socially anxious and shy with attention problems.

A number of clinical attributes are found commonly in those with ASCs that may complicate the communication of information and dialogue between client and counselor. These include

- Literal thinking and understanding
- One-sidedness
- Lack of empathy and understanding of others feelings
- Friendship and social difficulties
- Problems with meaning and use of language
- Obsessional preoccupations/behaviors
- Lack of imaginary play.

Any aspects of language that rely heavily on hidden meanings, metaphors, sarcasm, or irony will present difficulties, as will proverbs.

Attention Deficit-Hyperactivity Disorder

A range of twin, sibling, family, and adoption studies support a very strong genetic basis to this spectrum of disorders (Elia & Devoto 2007). Also, ADHD can be the presenting disorder for a range of genetic conditions, including fragile X syndrome (Turk 1998), Turner syndrome (Russell et al. 2006), Smith-Magenis syndrome, neurofibromatosis, tuberous sclerosis, and Williams syndrome (Lo-Castro, D'Agati, & Curatolo 2011).

Self-Injurious Behavior

Self-injurious behavior is a common, debilitating, serious, and difficult-to-treat complication of severe intellectual disability. The likelihood, intensity, frequency, and persistence of self-injury have substantial psychological underpinnings, with maladaptive learning and poor communication skills often being implicated (Arron, Oliver, Moss, Berg, & Burbidge 2011). However, the topography, or nature, of the self-injury seems to be highly genetically determined and specific to certain genetic conditions. For example, individuals with Lesch-Nyhan syndrome characteristically gnaw at their knuckles and bite their lips and hands, whereas those with Cornelia de Lange syndrome bite their lips and head bang. People with fragile X syndrome tend to bite themselves at the base of the thumb in response to excitement or anxiety. Prader-Willi syndrome produces gross overeating with associated morbid obesity, as well as a tendency to pick and scratch at the already delicate skin. Smith-Magenis syndrome produces a constellation of developmental challenges comprising intellectual disability, social and communicatory difficulties, severe sleep disturbance, marked attentional deficits, and severe self-injury in the form of head banging, hair pulling, nail pulling, and reportedly a tendency to insert objects into bodily orifices.

PREPARATION FOR THE CONSULTATION

The room should be calm, spacious, and nonthreatening. It should contain a range of developmentally appropriate toys and drawing equipment. Some children with developmental difficulties will want to join in the "grown-up" discussion, whereas others will prefer to play and occupy themselves, and both eventualities should be catered for.

Many children, given sufficiently clear and straightforward information, will benefit from the genetic counseling session. One should always assume that the child has the capacity and awareness to understand the consultation and the reasons for it. One should therefore include and engage the child in discussion, as well as offering the opportunity to ask questions and make comments. Providing genetic counseling to individuals with developmental disabilities will, as a rule, involve not only the client but also caregivers and other family members. Families will need to cope with the counseling information and implications for the client and also for themselves. The individual with developmental disabilities has as much right to know and understand the complex information as other people, and so efforts need to be made to provide the information in as clear and comprehensible a fashion as possible, while always involving and including the individual, presenting information in as accessible a form as possible, and providing information on useful support groups.

The capacity of the individual to understand the necessary information, if presented appropriately, should always be assumed. In preparation, and with the caregiver's (and, if possible, child's) agreement and consent, it will be useful to gather information from the range of services and sources relevant to the child. These will usually include child health and pediatric services, child and adolescent mental health services, and education and social services.

It is also important to ascertain the names of the child's key supporting clinicians in the community, so that clinic letters can be copied to all relevant people. The timings of consultations should, if possible, fit in with the family's schedule so as to impinge as little as possible on the school day and caregiver's work schedules. When the child is more learning disabled or shows markedly challenging behaviors, more time should be allocated to the session, and consideration given as to whether the caregivers should be met with alone, with the child being included possibly at a later date.

Home visits may sometimes be desirable in these respects, and it may be necessary to have two healthcare professionals present, one attending to the child to allow the other to talk with caregivers.

SUMMARY

A number of general principles can be applied to communicating with and counseling individuals who have intellectual disability, ASCs, or ADHD. These include

- Brief, clear, concrete bites of information
- Mindfulness of short concentration spans, exhaustion, anguish, and sense of guilt
- Time for information to be absorbed and considered
- Polite repetition
- Clear and simple written and pictorial information
- Information on relevant support groups
- Reality coupled with respect for individual's strengths and potential
- Information available for children and siblings, as well as for parents
- Repeat appointments
- Encouragement to use memory aids for queries
- Liaison with other relevant services: health, education, social, private and voluntary

RESOURCES

The most frequently useful United Kingdom websites will include:

- MENCAP: www.mencap.org.uk
- National Autistic Society: www.nas.org.uk
- ADD Information & Support Service: www.addiss.org.uk
- Down Syndrome Association: www.downs-syndrome.org.uk
- Fragile X Society: www.fragilex.org.uk

A wealth of information on other genetic conditions associated with developmental disabilities can be found through Contact-a-Family (www.cafamily.org.uk).

Arron, K., Oliver, C., Moss, J., Berg, K., & Burbidge, C. (2011). The prevalence and phenomenology of self-injurious and aggressive behaviour in genetic syndromes. *Journal of Intellectual Disability Research, 55*, 109–120.

Baieli, S., Pavone, L., Meli, C., Fiumara, A., & Coleman, M. (2003). Autism and phenylketonuria. *Journal of Autism & Developmental Disorders, 33*, 201–204.

Banaschewski, T., Coghill, D., Danckaerts, M., & Döpfner, M. (2009) *Attention-deficit hyperactivity disorder and hyperkinetic disorder.* Oxford, UK: Oxford University Press.

Baron-Cohen, S., Scott, F. J., Allison, C., Williams, J., Bolton, P., Matthews, F. E., et al . (2009). Prevalence of autism spectrum conditions: UK school-based population study. *British Journal of Psychiatry, 194*, 500–509.

Berney, T. P., Ireland, M., & Burn, J. (1999). Behavioural phenotype of Cornelia de Lange syndrome. *Archives of Disease in Childhood, 81*, 333–336.

Buelow, J. M., Austin, J. K., Perkins, S. M., Shen, J., Dunn, D. W., & Fastenau, P. S. (2003). Behaviour and mental health problems in children with epilepsy and low IQ. *Developmental Medicine & Child Neurology, 45*, 683–692.

Curatolo, P., Napolioni, V., & Moavero, R. (2010) Autism spectrum disorders in tuberous sclerosis: Pathogenetic pathways and implications for treatment. *Journal of Child Neurology, 25*, 873–880.

Elia, J., & Devoto, M. (2007). ADHD genetics: 2007 update. *Current Psychiatry Reports, 9*, 434–439.

Hall, S., Oliver, C., & Murphy, G. (2001). Self-injurious behaviour in young children with Lesch-Nyhan syndrome. *Developmental Medicine & Child Neurology, 43*, 745–749.

Howlin, P., Karpf, J., & Turk, J. (2005). Behavioural characteristics and autistic features in individuals with Cohen syndrome. *European Child & Adolescent Psychiatry, 14*, 57–64.

Johnson, H., Wiggs, L., Stores, G., & Huson, S. M. (2005). Psychological disturbance and sleep disorders in children with neurofibromatosis type 1. *Developmental Medicine & Child Neurology, 47*, 237–242.

Kumar, R. A., & Christian, S. L. (2009). Genetics of autism spectrum disorders. *Current Neurology & Neuroscience Reports, 9*, 188–197.

Leekam, S. R., Nieto, C., Libby, S. J., Wing, L., & Gould, J. (2007). Describing the sensory abnormalities of children and adults with autism. *Journal of Autism & Developmental Disorders, 37*, 894–910.

Lo-Castro, A., D'Agati, E., & Curatolo, P. (2011). ADHD and genetic syndromes. *Brain & Development, 33*, 456–461.

Losh, M., Adolphs, R., Poe, M. D., Couture, S., Penn, D., Baranek, G. T., et al . (2009). Neuropsychological profile of autism and the broad autism phenotype. *Archives of General Psychiatry, 66*, 518–526.

Matson, J. L., & Neale, D. (2009). Psychotropic medication use for challenging behaviours in persons with intellectual disabilities: an overview. *Research in Developmental Disabilities, 30*, 572–586.

McGuffin, P., & Rutter, M. (2002). Genetics of normal and abnormal development. In M. Rutter and E. Taylor (Eds.), *Child and adolescent psychiatry (pp. 185–204).* Oxford, UK: Blackwell Scientific Publications.

Merwood, A., & Asherson, P. (2011). Attention deficit hyperactivity disorder: A lifespan genetic perspective. *Advances in Mental Health & Intellectual Disabilities, 5*, 33–46.

Oliver, C., & Richards, C. (2010). Self-injurious behaviour in people with intellectual disability. *Current Opinion in Psychiatry, 23*, 412–416.

Oliver, C., Sloneem, J., Hall, S., & Arron, K. (2009). Self-injurious behaviour in Cornelia de Lange syndrome: 1. Prevalence and phenomenology. *Journal of Intellectual Disability Research, 53,* 575–589.

Parkes, J., White-Koning, M., Dickinson, H. O., Thyen, U., Arnaud, C., Beckung, E., et al. (2008). Psychological problems in children with cerebral palsy: A cross-sectional European study. *Journal of Child Psychology & Psychiatry, 49,* 405–413.

Piven, J., Palmer, P., Landa, R., Santangelo, S., Jacobi, D., & Childress, D. (1997). Personality and language characteristics in parents from multiple-incidence autism families. *American Journal of Medical Genetics (Neuropsychiatric Genetics), 74,* 398–411.

Plomin, R. (2008). *Behavioural genetics.* Worth Publishers.

Polanczyk, G., de Lima, M. S., Horta, B. L., Biederman, J., & Rohde, L. A. (2007). The world-wide prevalence of ADHD: A systematic review and meta-regression analysis. *American Journal of Psychiatry, 164,* 856–858.

Robey, K. L., Reck, J. F., Giacomini, K. D., Barabas, G., & Eddey, G. E. (2003). Modes and patterns of self-mutilation in persons with Lesch-Nyhan disease. *Developmental Medicine & Child Neurology, 45,* 167–171.

Russell, H. F., Wallis, D., Mazzocco, M. M. M., Moshang, T., Zackai, E., Zinn, A. R., et al. (2006). Increased prevalence of ADHD in Turner syndrome with no evidence of imprinting effects. *Journal of Pediatric Psychology, 31,* 945–955.

Shelley, B. P., & Robertson, M. M. (2005). The neuropsychiatry and multisystem features of the Smith-Magenis syndrome: A review. *Journal of Neuropsychiatry & Clinical Neuroscience, 17,* 91–97.

Swillen, A., Verhoeven, W., & Fryns, J. P. (2002). Prader-Willi syndrome: New insights in the behavioural and psychiatric spectrum. *Journal of Intellectual Disability Research, 46,* 41–50.

Turk, J. (1996). Working with parents of children who have severe learning disabilities. *Clinical Child Psychology & Psychiatry, 1,* 581–596.

Turk, J. (1998). Fragile X syndrome and attentional deficits. *Journal of Applied Research in Intellectual Disabilities, 11,* 175–191.

Turk, J. (2004). Children with developmental disabilities and their parents. In P. Graham (Ed.), *Cognitive behaviour therapy for children and families* (2nd ed., pp. 244–262). Cambridge, UK: Cambridge University Press.

Turk, J. (2007a). Chromosomal abnormalities. In S. Ayers, A. Baum, C. McManus, S. Newman, K. Wallston, J. Weinman, et al (Eds.), *Cambridge handbook of psychology, health and medicine* (2nd ed., pp. 625–629). Cambridge, UK: Cambridge University Press.

Turk, J. (2007b). Behavioural phenotypes: Their applicability to children and young people who have intellectual disability. *Advances in Mental Health in Learning Disabilities, 1,* 4–13.

Turk, J. (2011). Fragile X syndrome: Lifespan developmental implications for those without as well as with intellectual disability. *Current Opinion in Psychiatry, 24,* 387–397.

Turk, J., & Graham, P. (1997). Fragile X syndrome, autism and autistic features. *Autism, 1,* 175–197.

Turk, J., Graham, P. J., & Verhulst, F. (2007). *Child & adolescent psychiatry: A developmental approach* (4th ed.). Oxford, UK: Oxford University Press.

Turk, J., & O'Brien, G. (2002).Counselling parents & carers of individuals with behavioural phenotypes. In G. O'Brien (Ed.), *Behavioural phenotypes in clinical practice* (pp. 152–168). London: MacKeith Press.

Wing, L. (2003). *The autistic spectrum: A guide for parents and professionals.* London: Constable & Robinson.

10 Communicating with Clients Who Are Terminally Ill

Anna-Marie Stevens and Jayne Wood

Don't appear so scholarly, pray. Humanize your talk, and speak to be understood.
—*Moliere*

Effective communication is critical for the delivery of optimal medical care, irrespective of the clinical scenario or setting. Communicating information to the client with a diagnosis of a life-limiting illness, however, poses particular challenges. The client may be more likely to be in distress from physical, psychological, and/or spiritual causes, all of which may pose a barrier to effective communication and affect the ability of the client to engage in dialogue. In such situations, there is an increased need for the healthcare professional to be observant for nonverbal as well as verbal cues, to optimize the environment of the consultation, and to ensure support is available for the client both during the consultation and following it.

In this chapter, we focus on preparing and conducting the consultation with the terminally ill client, highlighting important aspects of the interaction that will facilitate delivery of information in a sensitive manner (see Box 10.1).

BACKGROUND

The terminally ill client attending the consultation may be seeking genetic information regarding the terminal illness itself or about a condition quite separate to it. Not unlike any other client attending the clinic, the client is likely to be concerned as to whether he or she has an inherited condition (or risk of), if so what the risk is to relatives or children. The End of Life Care Strategy (Department of Health 2008) indicates a priority for care at the end of life to ensure that all

Box 10.1 Case Study

Mrs. A was a 39-year-old woman with a diagnosis of metastatic breast cancer. The disease had spread to her bones and liver. It had been noted that her liver function tests were also deteriorating. Mrs. A had a family history of breast cancer. Her mother had bilateral breast cancer that metastasized to the bone, lung, and brain; she died aged 59. A maternal aunt diagnosed with breast cancer aged 76 was alive and well. A cousin (again on the maternal side) died from breast cancer at the age of 57. Mrs. A had an elder brother and sister both alive and well. She had always been aware of her family history of breast cancer but until now had not wished to explore it further. Mrs. A was married, with two children, both daughters aged 9 and 6.

On presentation at the gentic clinic Ms A looked anxious.

In whatever format the verbal communication takes place, it is essential to ensure the congruence of this with any nonverbal communication. How things are said is often as important as what is said (Jenkins et al. 2010).

The Consultation

On arrival, Mrs. A entered the room looking frail and anxious, and took a seat. Her husband had been unable to attend with her due to unexpected work commitments and thus she had attended alone. She had attended via hospital transport, and the journey had been rather uncomfortable. She described some mild abdominal discomfort (2/10 on the visual analogue scale for pain) but stated that generally her pain was well controlled with regular opioid analgesia commenced by the palliative care team in the community a week ago. On questioning how she was feeling and her understanding of her current situation, Mrs. A explained that she knew options for further conventional anticancer treatment were now no longer available in view of her deteriorating liver function and progressive disease. She was feeling increasingly fatigued and had not been out of the house over the past week, spending most of the time in bed. She became tearful and said that although she was not afraid for herself, she was worried about the effect her clinical condition was having on her young family and the implications for their future. Although she had initially declined genetic testing when first diagnosed, the change in her condition over the past few weeks had changed her view, and she now wished to explore the possibility. After having some time to recover, and being given the opportunity to return another time for the discussion if the present meeting was too difficult, Mrs. A expressed a keen desire to continue with the consultation. The process of genetic testing was explained to her at a pace comfortable for her. Frequent opportunities were given to allow her to ask questions and reflect on what was being said. To facilitate communication, notes were made so that she could take them away and share them with her husband. She was also keen to be copied into any letters that were being written to other professionals so that she might fully understand what was being said. She was asked how she would prefer the results to be given to her. She expressed that, although she would prefer to return to the gentic' clinic, the journey had been uncomfortable and she wasn't sure she would like to repeat it. She was asked how she would like to receive the results should she be unable to return to the clinic herself. To this she requested that she would like her husband to attend with her sister, who could then relay the information back to her. She had become very tired during the consultation and, at this point, stated that she had no further questions and would like to proceed with genetic testing.

Tips for the Consultation

- The client has previously not wished to discuss the issue of gentic; therefore, creating a relaxed reassuring atmosphere in the first few minutes of the consultation is important.
- Ensuring the environment for the consultation is comfortable and private for any client will be of pivotal importance in sharing any issues or concerns.
- For the client who is terminally ill, the questioning format of the consultation should be no different from any other consultation. A combination of open and closed questions should be used.
- The client may be thinking about the future and any impact discussing gentic will have on his or her children. Tolerate short silences. Silence usually means the client is feeling or thinking about something particularly significant. (Buckman 1994)

clients experience high-quality care irrespective of diagnosis. To date, much of the literature available explores the needs of clients at the end of life with a diagnosis of cancer, although it would seem fair to extend this evidence to those with a terminal illness secondary to a nonmalignant cause. The literature highlights the importance that clients and their caregivers place on good communication with their healthcare professionals.

The National Health Service (NHS) Cancer Plan (Department of Health 2000) suggests that although some cancer clients reported examples of excellent communication from staff, others reported the opposite, with information being delivered in a manner that failed to enable the client to feel adequately informed about his or her diagnosis and thus not feel able to contribute to the decision-making process about his or her management plan. Although communication may be through a variety of different means, most clients place high value on receiving information in a face-to-face consultation and expect it to be of high quality (National Institute for Clinical Excellence [NICE] 2004).

Cox et al. (2006) conducted a multicentered U.K. study evaluating multidisciplinary team communication. The information experiences of 394 cancer clients were audited: 87% wanted all possible information to be delivered, whether good or bad in nature and 39% of clients wanted to share responsibility for decision making. For this to happen, the client must be fully informed, which in turn relies upon good communication.

> Poor communication leads to dissatisfaction among patients, which can result in poor compliance with recommended treatments. Finally, it can lead to registered complaints (Department of Health 2000).

PREPARING FOR THE CONSULTATION

Preparing for the consultation with the terminally ill client should begin by anticipating questions that may arise and collating as much information as possible to be able to answer them. Sources of information might include a referral letter, medical notes, or discussion with other healthcare professionals, such as the referring clinician, general practitioner (GP), community palliative care team, or key worker such as a clinical nurse specialist.

Collecting family history information is a key part of assessing the genetic risk for the individual and his or her family. The client may not be well enough to complete a family history questionnaire prior to the appointment or may feel overwhelmed by the request. If the usual practice includes sending a family history questionnaire in advance of the appointment or with the appointment letter, it would be useful to also include a note explaining that this type of information is needed but reassuring the client that the practitioners can take the family history at the appointment and make an initial assessment with limited information. It may be useful to suggest that a relative helps to provide the information.

> The decision as to where to conduct the consultation is likely to depend on the health and emotional status of the client. Ideally, the consultation should take place in a quiet room, away from interruptions, but it may be appropriate to consider a home visit to minimize discomfort.

Many clients prefer to be accompanied (e.g., by family, caregiver, friend, or key worker) to consultations, particularly when delivery of sensitive information is anticipated. Clients should be offered this option when arranging the appointment so that the cleint can make arrangements to be accompanied, and the clinician can make arrangements for additional people to be present (e.g., bringing in additional chairs, ensuring that everyone knows where exactly to meet and where, if driving, to park).

When booking the appointment and informing the client, be mindful of any disability that the client may have, secondary to disease or otherwise, that may affect his or her ability to write or remember the information being shared, . It may be worth ensuring, with the consent of the client, that someone else also knows about the appointment (e.g., family, caregiver, key worker, and/or GP).

COMMUNICATION IN THE CONSULTATION

At the first consultation, address the referral letter issued by the referring health-care professional, outlining the clinical picture and any family history information collected prior to the appointment. It is important to establish what the client understands of his or her diagnosis and current clinical condition early on in the consultation. This may differ from what is written in his or her medical notes. Collation of this information makes it not only possible to learn the client's perspective, but also allows identification of language familiar to the client and allows the practitioner to pick up on cues regarding the client's feelings and coping strategies. This may inform how further information is delivered and what future support might be appropriate.

As with any genetic counseling session, it is important to check the client's understanding of why he or she has been referred, what will happen at the appointment, and what the client's agenda is for the appointment. Once the presenting history has been ascertained, the history taking should proceed as normal, being mindful of the holistic approach and paying particular attention to the assessment of psychological, social, and spiritual needs.

> Taking family history information can be emotionally challenging, especially if recounting details of relatives who have died prematurely from the presumed genetic illness. For the terminally ill client, this can be particularly poignant, so it is important to be aware of his or her responses and feelings and be flexible about how much detail you collect about the family history during the consultation.

If a physical examination is required, it is important to identify any symptoms that the client may be experiencing such as pain, nausea, and vomiting to minimize discomfort caused by the assessment.

> If the referral for a genetic assessment is for a client who is at the end of life, it will have to be dealt with urgently. There may be a need to conduct the consultation by phone or at the bedside on the ward or in the hospice, and there may not be an opportunity for a follow-up appointment.

When counseling clients at the end of life, it is important to obtain a blood sample to store DNA, if a decision for testing cannot immediately be made. Obtain details of an alternative contact person(s), so the implications of the genetic assessment can be cascaded to the at-risk relatives, even after the client's death. It can feel challenging to ask the client for this information and acknowledge that the genetic issues may be a legacy for his or her family, after death. Clients may feel distressed by this or they may feel relieved that they have helped their family by seeing the gentic doctor and giving a sample of blood so that testing can be undertaken to inform the risk of relatives.

The closure of the consultation should consist of a summary of information exchanges between the healthcare professional and client, being sure to prioritize concerns raised by the client. Time must be given to allow the client to ask questions and for a management plan to be discussed and made. Ideally, the client should be given a future appointment, especially if the information exchanged was in any way distressing to him or her. If this is not possible or appropriate for any reason, the client should be given contact details in the event that he or she has further questions or needs further support. If testing is to be undertaken, the client needs to be informed of the likely timescale and plans made for disseminating the results. Finally, the consultation should be well documented and details of alternate contact and consent clearly included in the notes. When documenting the consultation in a letter, try to avoid putting in new information that wasn't discussed with the client. Many clients now receive copies of these clinic letters, and for them to receive new information in this way can be very distressing.

Verbal and Nonverbal Cues

Some aspects of communication in terms of verbal and nonverbal behavior may be demonstrated by the healthcare professional and the client which, once recognized, may facilitate good communication by not only gathering more information but also in the development of a rapport between the two individuals. This is particularly important when considering clients in distress, such as those with a terminal illness, who may be much less able and willing to engage in open discussion.

The use of language may vary according to what is familiar to the client; this may in turn be influenced by cultural beliefs. Where possible, and certainly at the beginning of the consultation, the questions should be open, allowing the client to offer as much information as possible and preventing the client from feeling as though there is a strict agenda that he or she should not move away from.

In circumstances when the client's first language is not that of the healthcare professional, a professional interpreter should be arranged. The highly sensitive nature of information being exchanged between the healthcare professional and the terminally ill client makes the commonplace practice of using a nonprofessional interpreter, often in the form of a family member or caregiver, ill-advised unless unavoidable. The client may feel unable to be open in discussing sensitive issues, and the nonprofessional interpreter may filter information to the client to minimize distress.

Barriers to Effective Communication

Barriers that may be encountered when communicating with the terminally ill client may be initiated by the healthcare professional or by the client. Being aware of such elements facilitates the healthcare professional to be able to identify and work through them.

The healthcare professional may avoid open discussion for fear of upsetting the client, or causing more harm than good and unleashing strong emotions that he or she may feel unable to deal with. He or she may be concerned that the client will ask difficult, unanswerable questions, and that, in attempting to answer them, he or she may say the wrong thing and cause more distress.

The client may avoid open discussion if he or she is unsure of the agenda of the meeting and the role of the healthcare professional present. He or she may be concerned that talking about his or her suffering may not be welcomed and may simply increase the burden on the healthcare professional.

Clients may exhibit specific behaviors that avoid topics raised by the healthcare professional. Examples are "blocking," in which the client moves the interviewer away from a particular topic that he or she does not wish to discuss, and "switching focus," in which the client picks up on part of the content of what the interviewer has said but steers it away from particular aspects of the topic that he or she doesn't wish to discuss.

In response to blocking and switching behaviors, the healthcare professional should avoid common pitfalls in responding, such as giving premature or false reassurance, of using medical jargon, and of normalizing the client experience, which, although it may be reassuring for the client, may detract from his or her individual experience.

The consultation by the genetic healthcare professional, as with any consultation, may have a well-defined agenda. However, it is quite possible that topics discussed may evoke an emotional response, thus forcing the consultation down a quite different route to that initially embarked upon and requiring the healthcare professional to perform a more holistic assessment that the non–palliative care specialist may or may not feel confident at performing.

A holistic assessment should be ongoing for a client, but it should also be structured around certain time points, including any time a client requests and around the time of diagnosis (NICE 2004). Delivery of new genetic information may add a further layer of information to the understanding a client may have of his or her diagnosis, thus prompting a need for further review of the client's needs.

SUMMARY

- Guidance is available on the delivery of optimal care for the client with a terminal illness and who is at the end of life.
- Clients with a terminal illness are likely to have symptoms that may be of a physical, psychological, and/or spiritual nature, which may pose a barrier to effective communication.
- When preparing for the consultation, consider:

  - The location of the consultation and environment
  - Who should be present
  - When it should happen
  - Assistance with transport if necessary
  - Who should be aware of it
  - Adjustments that might need to be made to accommodate any disability

- During the consultation:

  - Be attentive to nonverbal cues to facilitate communication.
  - Use open rather than closed questions to gain information.
  - Be prepared to holistically assess symptoms so that appropriate support can be offered subsequently.
  - Ensure that the client is allowed ample opportunity to ask questions and that information is delivered in manageable portions.
  - Close the consultation by summarizing information exchanges and discussing a management plan.

- After the consultation, ensure that documentation of the discussion is clear and communicated with other relevant individuals.

REFERENCES

Buckman, R. (1994). *How to break bad news: A guide for health care professionals*. London: Papermac.

Cox, A., Jenkins, V., Catt, S., Langridge, V., & Fallowfield, L. (2006). Information needs and experiences: An audit of cancer patients. *European Journal of Oncology Nursing, 10*, 263–272.

Department of Health. (2000). *The NHS cancer plan*. London: Author. Accessed March 14, 2011 from http://www.dh.gov.uk/prod_consum_dh/groups/dh_digitalassets/@dh/@en/documents/digitalasset/dh_4014513.pdf

Department of Health. (2008). *End of life care strategy—Promoting high quality care for all adults at the end of life*. London: Author. Accessed March 14, 2011from http://www.dh.gov.uk/prod_consum_dh/groups/dh_digitalassets/@dh/@en/documents/digitalasset/dh_086345.pdf

Health Care Commission. (2007). *State of healthcare 2007*. London: Author. Accessed March 14, 2011 from http://www.official-documents.gov.uk/document/hc0708/hc00/0097/0097.pdf

Jenkins, V., Farewell, D., Batt, L., Maughan, T., Branston, L., Langridge, C., et al. (2010). The attitudes of 1066 patients with cancer towards participation in randomised clinical trials. *British Journal of Cancer, 103*(12), 1801–1807.

National Cancer Action Team. (2008). *Connected national communication skills training participant handbook—Advanced communication skills*. Accessed February 24, 2012 from http://www.connected.nhs.uk

National Institute for Clinical Excellence (NICE). (2004). *Supportive and palliative care for people with cancer*. Accessed March 14, 2011from http://www.nice.org.uk/nicemedia/live/10893/28816/28816.pdf

11 Communicating with Clients Who Have Dementia

Rachel Taylor

Identification is one of the key ingredients of effective communication. In fact, unless your listeners can identify with what you are saying and with the way you are saying it, they are not likely to receive and understand your message.
—Hema Ravi

Dementia is caused by a number of different diseases and conditions. It is therefore not a single diagnosis but rather a complex syndrome that is associated with a progressive decline in multiple areas of function including memory, reasoning, judgement, planning, language, communication, and understanding. It also impairs a person's ability to carry out daily activities and is strongly associated with behavioral and psychological symptoms. It is estimated that there are currently more than 700,000 people with dementia living in the United Kingdom (Department of Health 2009), and recent figures from the U.S. Alzheimer's Association show that around 5.4 million Americans are currently diagnosed with dementia (Alzheimer's Association 2011).

The most common cause of dementia is Alzheimer's disease, and the exact cause or causes of this are still unknown, although most experts agree that there are probably a number of contributing factors. At present, a genetic cause of dementia has only been identified in a minority of conditions, perhaps the most well known of which is Huntington's disease; therefore, the number of people who have dementia with a known genetic cause is relatively small. However, the discovery of further causative genes is ongoing, and genetic risk, whether it has been identified or not, is a cause of great concern to many affected people and their families (Wild & Tabrizi 2007).

Expert opinion in the field is that diagnostic genetic testing in people with dementia should only be carried out on the basis of clinical likelihood and only then following genetic counseling (Knopman et al. 2001). However, the very nature of the problems that people with dementia experience can make the genetic counseling of symptomatic clients challenging.

The aim of this chapter is to offer some hints and guidance to genetic professionals to assist them in effectively engaging and communicating with individuals with dementia, to enable them to ensure that, when possible, information is given in an appropriate manner that best facilitates the individual's understanding and decision making.

BACKGROUND

A person with dementia might present for genetic counseling for three main reasons:

- The cause of his or her dementia is likely to be genetic, based on clinical signs and symptoms and/or family history, and genetic testing is being considered by the clinical team.
- The individual and/or his or her family may be concerned that his or her dementia has a genetic cause and so wish to discuss this and the potential risks to family members.
- The individual with dementia may be at risk of another unrelated inherited condition and so may request or be referred for genetic counseling.

Genetic Causes of Dementia

The majority of cases of dementia are not due to a clearly identifiable genetic cause, and the genes that are known to cause dementia are very rare in the general population (Wild & Tabrizi 2007). The mode of inheritance for Huntington's disease is well documented and straightforward. However, by comparison, in Alzheimer's disease, only about 3% of cases have onset of symptoms before 60 years of age, and, of these cases, around 60% are familial, 13% of which show clear autosomal dominant inheritance (Campion et al. 1999). Even in the presence of a family history of dementia, factors such as misdiagnosis, clinical heterogeneity, phenocopies, and early death due to other causes can make it very difficult to establish a clear mode of inheritance (Quaid 2011).

Some of the identified genetic causes of dementia include mutations in the following genes: *PSEN1* and *PSEN2* (early-onset autosomal dominant Alzheimer's disease), *MAPT* (frontotemporal dementia), *HTT* (Huntington's disease), *PRNP* (familial prion disease), and *Notch3* (CADASIL—cerebral autosomal dominant arteriopathy with subcortical infarcts and leukoencephalopathy, an inherited vascular dementia). See www.genetests.org for more in-depth information on the genetic causes of dementia.

Symptoms in Dementia

To start thinking about how best to work with an individual who has a diagnosis of dementia, it is helpful to be aware of the sorts of symptoms and problems he or she may be experiencing. The Alzheimer's Society produces some very useful factsheets that can be downloaded from its website www.alzheimers.org.uk. Most people think of memory loss as the main symptom in dementia and although most dementias involve some degree of memory loss, some forms do not, especially in the early stages. Other areas that can be affected are personality and behavior, reasoning, and language and perceptual skills, but the particular difficulties an individual has will be dependent on a number of factors, including the type of dementia and disease stage. Some of the more common symptoms that individuals may experience, which may be of particular relevance for genetic counseling, include:

- *Memory*: Short-term memory in particular is often impaired and so people can easily forget recent conversations and events and find it difficult to retain new information. They will often misplace items and forget important dates, such as birthdays. They may have trouble remembering names and places and find themselves getting lost on once familiar journeys or in familiar places. Disorientation to time and place is a fairly common problem for people with Alzheimer's disease but less so for people with Huntington's disease, for example. Semantic memory (i.e., the ability to store facts and knowledge about the world) is pretty well preserved in people with Huntington's disease (although it may be impaired due to other problems associated with the condition); however, loss of conceptual knowledge is a common feature in cortical dementias such as Alzheimer's disease (Craufurd & Snowden 2002). Studies have shown that people at comparative stages of Huntington's disease and Alzheimer's disease perform equally poorly on free recall when given a list learning task; however, individuals with Huntington's disease do much better when they are given cues to remind them or when encouraged to use word association (Craufurd & Snowden 2002; Pillon, Deweer, Agid, & Dubois 1993).
- *Communication and understanding*: In addition to physical problems with verbal communication, such as dysarthria, many people with dementia experience difficulties with language in that they have trouble finding the right words for things, and they may either substitute an incorrect word or not find any word at all. This is a particularly prevalent problem for people with cortical dementias, and it can result in incomprehensible sentences and phrases and cause a great deal of frustration for affected individuals and their caregivers. Language in people with Huntington's disease is relatively well preserved but communication becomes increasingly impaired due to the progressive motor impairment. It is important to encourage a person with dementia to communicate in the way that he or she finds easiest, and awareness of nonverbal means of communication such as gestures, touch, and facial expressions becomes more important.

Lack of initiative and apathy, which are also common features of many forms of dementia, can make it difficult for people to start a conversation or ask a question, and many people find it difficult to respond to open-ended questions. People with dementia may also have a greatly slowed response time. As dementia progresses, clients find it increasingly difficult to understand new information or concepts and to communicate thoughts and decisions.

- *Personality and behavior*: People with dementia can often exhibit significant personality and behavioral changes, and they may become more aggressive, irritable, anxious, suspicious, and confused. Repetitive behavior is common, and many people will "get stuck" on asking the same question over and over again or repeating the same phrase or action. People with dementia can also experience restlessness, and they may pace up and down because of this or because they want something but are unable to express what they want. People with dementia may become disinhibited and say and/or do things that are inappropriate; this can be a particular problem for people with frontotemporal lobe dementia. Mood changes are also common, particularly low mood and depression. Additionally, people can exhibit rapid mood changes, for example, going from calm to angry to tearful in a short space of time with no apparent trigger. They are also often very sensitive to overstimulation (e.g., too much noise or crowded places with lots of people).

- *Reasoning and judgment*: Executive function (i.e., the cognitive ability to plan, organize, and problem solve) is affected in most forms of dementia. Clients find it very difficult to concentrate on or do more than one thing at once and, even early on in the course of their disease, they can be easily distracted and lose their train of thought. Lack of insight and denial can be problematic, particularly in Huntington's disease. People can exhibit poor judgment, and their behavior can be impulsive as they find it difficult to consider the consequences of their actions. Weighing up information in order to make a decision becomes very difficult and this, combined with problems understanding and retaining information, has a major impact on individuals' capacity to make a decision for themselves (see Mental Capacity Act [Department for Constitutional Affairs 2005]: Code of Practice, for further helpful information).

PREPARING FOR THE CONSULTATION

Attending a hospital outpatient clinic appointment can be a stressful and worrying event for anyone. It can be particularly difficult for people with dementia as it usually involves a change to their routine; a significant journey; an often unfamiliar, busy, and noisy environment; and new faces.

A home visit may be preferable, certainly for a first appointment, as the person may feel more comfortable and less stressed in his or her home environment; this may have a beneficial effect on communication, memory, and mood. If a home visit is a possibility, it would be helpful to speak with the person or loved one, friend, or caregiver on their behalf beforehand to find out how this would work practically and to try and ensure that someone will be with the person at the visit. If that will be impossible or the person doesn't have someone who can be there, it is advisable to think about arranging to do the visit with someone that the person is familiar with, for example a family doctor, social worker, or visiting nurse.

Prior to the genetic team seeing the person with dementia, it may be useful to seek further advice from a professional with expertise, such as a specialist nurse for dementia. Their guidance and input can be invaluable, and, if appropriate, they may also be able to attend the appointment, although the usefulness of this should be balanced with the potential distress caused by increasing numbers of people at the consultation.

Additionally, having background information about the individual is extremely useful in planning the consultation. Knowing the sorts of symptoms they have and how long they have had these symptoms is helpful, and this information can be obtained from the individual, his or her family or caregivers, and professionals involved in his or her care, such as a general practitioner, psychiatrist, neurologist, or specialist nurse. The results of cognitive assessments done by psychologists can also enable the genetic professional to appropriately plan ahead.

Clinic Booking

The appointment booking process should be as simple as possible. It is important to consider that some people with dementia don't open their mail or may misplace appointment letters. Thus, arranging the appointment by telephone with either the individual or a loved one, friend, or caregiver may be more appropriate. Although respecting the individual's autonomy and confidentiality, it can sometimes be too overwhelming and/or confusing for someone with dementia to arrange a hospital appointment, and so, if appropriate, it can be useful to establish whether there is someone the client booking team can liaise with on behalf of the client. If making the appointment over the telephone with the person with dementia, he or she should be encouraged to put the appointment on a calendar or in a diary if he or she uses those things as memory aids. A reminder telephone call close to the appointment can also be helpful, as can text messages or e-mails (if appropriate and used by the individual or his or her designated contact).

The time of day of the appointment is also worth considering as some people with dementia may be more alert and less confused at certain times of day. This may correspond to timing of medication, how tired the individual is, and whether his or her sleep pattern is altered.

It is also important to consider how the individual will get to the appointment. Although some people will be physically able to travel on public transport, others may not, either because they have physical symptoms that impair their mobility and/or because they find traveling on public transport too overwhelming and confusing. It may be that, in some cases, hospital client transport is required, and it can be useful to liaise directly with hospital transport services, if they are available. Otherwise some charitable organizations may be able to provide transport.

The Waiting Area

A busy, noisy waiting room is not an ideal place for most people with dementia. By planning in advance with reception staff, it may be possible to arrange for the person to wait in a quieter area if one is available. If the person is restless or agitated, he or she may prefer to wait outside. If he or she or their escort have a mobile telephone, and it is safe for them to wait outside, reception staff can call when they are due to be seen.

Timing of Consultations

The amount of time needed for the appointment will depend on the individual. Someone in the earlier stages of dementia may require a longer appointment so that information can be given slowly and repeated, and to allow him or her time to both answer and ask questions. If he or she is with family members, the likelihood is that they will want to ask questions also. However many people with dementia will find it difficult to concentrate for long periods, and their attention will be significantly reduced. Therefore, it may be that shorter appointments are easier for them to manage and arrangements can be made to speak with family members separately.

COMMUNICATION IN THE CONSULTATION

Understanding and Decision Making

Genetic counseling is traditionally concerned with imparting information with the intention of enabling decision making (see Box 11.1). For some people with very early dementia, it may be relatively straightforward to ascertain that the individual has understood and retained the information and used it to make a decision that he or she has clearly communicated. For others, it will be clear that they do not have capacity to make that specific decision (e.g., whether to have genetic testing or not) because they haven't understood, retained, and processed the information given to them. However, this can be a difficult assessment for genetic professionals to make. In these complex cases, the input from other relevant healthcare professionals in the process, such as a dementia specialist (neurologist or specialist nurse), psychiatrist, and/or psychologist, is crucial. The thoughts and feelings of family members, loved ones, and/or friends are important, particularly if a "best interests" decision will be

Box 11.1 Tips for Communicating with Someone with Dementia

The following tips are based on guidance from the Alzheimer's Society (www.alzheimers.org.uk) and the Huntington's Disease Association (www.hda.org.uk). Both organizations produce helpful information regarding communication, which can be downloaded from their websites. Many of these tips will sound familiar to genetic professionals as they involve strategies that they utilize regularly in their everyday practice.

Listening

- Listen carefully to what the person is saying, giving him or her encouragement but also being careful not to interrupt unless necessary. It is important to be patient as it takes longer for the brain of a person with dementia to process information, and responses are slowed.
- If the person has trouble finding the right word, ask him or her to explain in a different way, if he or she is able.
- If the person's speech is difficult to understand, the person/people who know him or her best can be very helpful. Also using what you already know about the person can help in interpreting what he or she is saying. However, it is important to check back with the individual that you are correct—don't pretend to understand when you do not.
- Encourage the use of any communication aids that the person may normally use.
- Use cues and guidance where appropriate.
- If the person moves off topic, sensitively refocus him or her. If a person gets stuck on a topic or phrase, gently making him or her aware of this can be helpful. Allowing time on a particular topic before moving onto another can be useful, as can informing the person that the subject or topic is changing.
- If the person gets upset or sad, allow him or her to express feelings.

Speaking

- Speak clearly and calmly, using a reduced rate of speech; avoid raising your voice.
- Use simple, short sentences.
- Avoid asking open-ended or direct questions in which the person may struggle to find the answer. Questions that allow a yes or no response or either/or questions allow the person more time to communicate his or her thoughts without the need for him or her to formulate a response.
- Repeat the message. However, it is also important to realize that if the message has been repeated several times, and the person is still not able to understand, another strategy should be used to prevent frustration.

(continued)

Box 11.1 (Continued)

- Saying something in a slightly different way can sometimes be helpful.
- Keep messages simple and try not to ask the person to make complicated choices.
- Sometimes spelling a key word can be helpful.
- Recognize that the person with dementia may not be able to initiate a conversation.
- Be wary of patronizing the person and, if you are getting little response from him or her, avoid speaking about him or her as if he or she isn't there, as this can cause considerable distress to the individual.

Body Language

- Use facial expressions and gestures as a means of communication, picking up cues from the individual's body language.
- Be aware of your own body language—a tense facial expression, for example, may cause the person to become upset.
- Be calm, still, and relaxed—never stand over someone to communicate. Rather, sit at their level, make eye contact, and be aware of personal space.

Environment

- Minimize distractions and background noise as much as possible.
- Where possible, optimize the temperature of the room and consider things like lighting and seating. Sitting behind a desk could be seen as threatening to the person with dementia.

Written Information

- Any written information given to the individual at the consultation or afterwards should be simple and easy to read.
- Jargon should be avoided.
- Simple pictures and diagrams can be helpful

Other Factors

- Check that if the person uses a hearing aid, it is working properly, and if he or she wears glasses, that these are available.
- Being aware of factors that may affect communication—such as pain, illness, fatigue, hunger, thirst, and side effects of medications—is helpful. If, for example, the person with dementia has an infection just prior to the planned appointment, this may exacerbate his or her symptoms and make communication and understanding even more difficult; it may be wise to reschedule the appointment.

made on behalf of a person who lacks capacity. The person's past wishes should be considered. If the individual is "unbefriended" (i.e., they do not have capacity to make a decision regarding genetic testing and they do not have family or friends who are appropriate to consult), then an Independent Mental Capacity Advocate (IMCA) should be consulted (for more information, see www.scie.org.uk/publications/imca/index.asp).

SUMMARY

- A person with dementia may request or be referred for genetic counseling either due to the potential inherited nature of the cause of his or her dementia or because he or she is at risk of another unrelated inherited condition.
- An awareness of the sorts of symptoms that a person with dementia might have allows the genetic professional to appropriately plan for consultations.
- Input from the person, his or her loved ones and/or caregivers, and professionals involved in his or her care is useful to ensure that consultations are pitched at the correct level for that individual.
- Being aware of tips and strategies to optimize communication with the person with dementia is crucial.

FURTHER READING

Clayton, H., Graham, N., Warner, J. (2010). *Alzheimer's and Other Dementias (answers at your fingertips)* (3rd edition). London: Class Publishing

The Mental Capacity Act (UK) 2005 [Pdf] Accessed from: http://www.legislation.gov.uk/ukpga/2005/9/pdfs/ukpga_20050009_En.pdf http://www.mencap.org.uk/sites/default/files/documents/2010–12/Comms_guide_dec_10.pdf

FOR FURTHER INFORMATION ABOUT ALZHEIMER'S DISEASE

In the United Kingdom: www.alzheimers.org.uk
In the United States: www.alz.org

FOR FURTHER INFORMATION ABOUT HUNTINGTON'S DISEASE

In the United Kingdom: www.hda.org.uk
In the United States: www.hdsa.org

REFERENCES

Alzheimer's Association. (2011). Alzheimer's disease facts and figures. *Alzheimer's and Dementia, 7*(2), 13–31.

Campion, D., Dumanchin, C., Hannequin, D., Dubois, B., Belliard, S., Puel, M., et al. (1999). Early-onset autosomal dominant Alzheimer disease: Prevalence, genetic heterogeneity, and mutation spectrum. *American Journal of Human Genetics, 65,* 664–670.

Craufurd, D., & Snowden, J. (2002). Neuropsychological and neuropsychiatric aspects of Huntington's disease. In G. Bates, P. Harper, & L. Jones (Eds.), *Huntington's disease* (3rd ed., pp. 62–94). Oxford, UK: Oxford University Press.

Department for Constitutional Affairs. (2007). *Mental Capacity Act 2005.Code of practice.* London: TSO.

Department of Health. (2009). *Living well with dementia: A national dementia strategy.* London: TSO.

Knopman, D. S., DeKosky, S. T., Cummings, J. L., Chui, H., Corey-Bloom, J., Relkin, N., et al. (2001). Practice parameter: Diagnosis of dementia (an evidence-base review): Report of the Quality Standards Subcommittee of the American Academy of Neurology. *Neurology, 56,* 1143–1153.

Pillon, B., Deweer, B., Agid, Y., & Dubois, B. (1993). Explicit memory in Alzheimer's, Huntington's, and Parkinson's diseases. *Archives of Neurology, 5 0*(4), 374–379.

Quaid, K. A. (2011). Genetic counseling for frontotemporal dementias. *Journal of Molecular Neuroscience, 45*(3),706–709.

Wild, E., & Tabrizi, S. (2007). Genetic causes of dementia. *Advances in Clinical Neuroscience and Rehabilitation, 7*(2), 14–16.

12 Communication from an Interpreter's Perspective

Nicki Cornwell

It is impossible to speak in such a way that you cannot be misunderstood.
—Karl Popper

As a French-speaking interpreter, my services have been used by a number of different health professionals. Sometimes the communication process was hampered by lack of knowledge and awareness on the part of the health professional as to how best to work with the interpreter. In this chapter, I suggest ways in which interpreters might be used effectively.

I begin by analyzing what makes for good communication between health professionals and clients, and I then go on to examine the effect of using a foreign language interpreter on the communication process. I have included two case studies: one of good practice and one of practice which was, at best, indifferent. I finish with pointers for good practice for working with an interpreter.

MY OWN PERSPECTIVES

I am a white British woman with a background in social work; my first language is English, my second is French. In the city in which I live, the influx of asylum seekers and refugees from French-speaking parts of Africa has resulted in an unprecedented demand for French interpreters. I thus took up employment as an interpreter. My services were requested and paid for by health and local authority departments. I therefore came into contact with a range of professionals and the users of their services.

As an interpreter, I had no responsibility for what was said or how it was said to me; only for transforming words from one language to another and relaying what was being said from one person to the other. I had an unparalleled opportunity to observe and reflect upon the interaction of professionals and those who use their services, and the communication between them. I also suffered a certain amount of frustration when I encountered professionals who were uncertain of how to make effective use of an interpreter.

In exploring what makes for effective use of an interpreter, I begin by analyzing what makes for good communication between professionals and the users of their services. I shall discuss elements of bridge-building between professionals and their clients: creating conditions for two-way traffic, checking the language that is used, aspects of power, and the importance of giving information about the agency and the services that are offered.

BUILDING A BRIDGE BETWEEN PROFESSIONAL AND CLIENT

In an initial contact with a client, professionals try to build a bridge between themselves and the client that is strong enough to carry communications both ways. If either lacks confidence that the structure is sound, communication will be subject to misconceptions and misinterpretation. Professionals have an agenda to carry out, according to the demands of their role, and what they hope for is the development of trust between themselves and the client. In building a sound bridge, the following are key elements of the communication process:

Two-way traffic: A genuine interest in hearing the client's point of view needs to be indicated, and a demonstrated ability to listen. It is vital to the communication process that the bridge that is built can carry traffic both ways.

Language and the use of jargon: Lay people find it difficult to understand incomprehensible medical language. Health professionals have a responsibility for decoding medical jargon, and, when they do so, they are acting as interpreters between themselves and other English-speaking people: thus interpretation does not always involve a foreign language. Health professionals also need to be flexible in the language that they use. They will have some clients with a poor command of spoken English, and others who may be more adept at expressing themselves than the professional. Other factors may affect communication: for example, if a person has learning disabilities, mental health problems, or problems with literacy.

Aspects of power in professional/client communication: There is no getting away from the fact that there is an imbalance of power between professionals and clients. Not only are health professionals perceived by clients as having power, but in reality they do have it. Health professionals have access to personal information about the client, they dictate the terms and conditions of accessing the health service, and they are a gatekeeper for access to other resources and services. Ways of minimizing the effects have been well charted: working in partnership, the use of negotiation, providing access to information and advice, and seeking to empower clients while being prepared to be an advocate when it is appropriate. These are all client-centered ways of working that are familiar to genetic counselors.

Other aspects of power should be considered. Any interaction between two people involves what sociologists refer to as *social positioning*. Each person sizes up the other in terms of race, culture, age, gender, and class, and takes up position in relation to the other in accordance with unspoken assumptions about underlying social hierarchies of inferiority and superiority. Social positioning can have an interference effect on professional–client communication, both by affecting the assumptions that professionals make about their clients, and the assumptions that clients make about professionals. Such assumptions can have powerful collusive effect: for example, a white couple might be uneasy about advice offered by a black professional, an older couple might be unwilling to accept advice given by a young professional, or there could be gender collusion between a male professional and a male client, or between a female professional and a female client. Professionals who are unaware of social positioning can unwittingly collude with inequalities of gender and race and the like.

GIVING INFORMATION ABOUT THE ROLE OF THE HEALTH PROFESSIONAL AND THE ROLE OF THE INTERPRETER

My experience of interpreting suggests that health professionals often fail to pay enough attention to the need to explain their role and that of the interpreter. What is clear to a professional is often far from clear to a client, who may be left very confused about what a professional can offer.

Each client has his or her own perspective on health services and on health professionals, grounded not only in differing cultural beliefs but also in his or her previous experiences of other professionals; clients also have their own views about the problems that they face and the help they need, and these perspectives may differ from those of the health professional. If there is no room for negotiation of these differences, and the client's perspective is swamped or can only be expressed as a form of conflict, communication between professional and user is not likely to be productive. It is therefore very important for the healthcare professional to give clear information about his or her role, the purpose of the consultation, and what he or she expects to discuss in the consultation (e.g., genetic risk assessment and a client's options for screening and testing, as appropriate). This can help to allay client's worries and set expectations at the appropriate level. The healthcare professional should also check the client's expectations for the appointment to ensure any discrepancy is revealed at the beginning of the session, so the client is not left feeling confused or dissatisfied. Finally, professionals need to have confidence in themselves and in their role; in the absence of confidence, how can trust develop? For examples of good and poor communication, see Boxes 12.1 and 12.2.

Box 12.1 Case Study 1

Marie-Louise was a refugee from a troubled African country. I was the interpreter for her initial visit to a general practitioner (GP), in which she complained about pain in her elbows and pain in her ankles. The GP made a diagnosis, suggested treatment, and told her to come back if things didn't improve.

On her third visit to the clinic, during which no improvement had been made, she happened to see a different GP; once again, I happened to be the interpreter. The doctor pursued the outcomes of the treatment that his colleague had offered. Then he said thoughtfully: "Are you under any stress at home?"

Yes, there was stress, she admitted. She was not very forthcoming, and the doctor could have left it at that; but he persevered with his questions.

"What kind of stress?"

"Housing and financial."

"Anything else?"

"I don't sleep very well."

Again, that could have been the end of the matter, but the doctor, a gentle and sensitive practitioner, was not satisfied.

"Have you got things on your mind, things that worry you?" he asked.

Little by little, he drew out a horrific tale of murder, rape, and eventual escape from a war-torn country. At last, he suggested that the complaint that she had come to discuss was the least of the problems facing her, and he offered to refer her to specialized services for the victims of war.

Box 12.2 Case Study 2

The next case study is in three parts. The unfortunate Celeste had two encounters involving indifferent professional practice, but an administrator did much to put matters right.

Celeste and the Visiting Nurse

Celeste was a recently arrived refugee from Africa; she and her lively 4-year-old son were living in temporary accommodation. A visiting nurse made a routine visit. The child was exuberant, but Celeste herself was quietly hesitant, impassive. She was living by herself, she said. She was possibly shy, possibly traumatized.

(continued)

Box 12.2 (Continued)

The visiting nurse ran through a list of questions about the child's medical history. Questions about the child's father (his family's medical history) met with reluctance, a shaking of shoulders, a stone-walling, yet the visiting nurse persisted in spite of the client's apparent reluctance to answer. I felt distaste at being obliged to relay her questions. I wanted to remind the visiting nurse that she was speaking to a refugee. Did she have no comprehension of the kind of experiences that might have driven Celeste to leave her country and seek refuge in the United Kingdom?

Celeste and the Consultant

My services had been requested by a consultant gynecologist in an outpatients' clinic. As I sat down beside the woman for whom I had come to interpret and introduced myself, I realized that I had seen her before. It's always difficult when that happens. You talk, you try not to drop any bricks, and all the time you are trying to dig up the details in your memory.

Where was it? I'm sure she was pregnant, I thought. Yet there was no sign of pregnancy now. She had an appointment with a gynecologist, but not in the maternity department. What had happened? Slowly the details came back to me. This was the Celeste I had interpreted for a visiting nurse, and subsequently I had helped a midwife to book her in for her scans. As I sat there, trying to pin down what was left of these memories, Celeste turned to me. She put her hand on her womb and said something. I hardly caught the words, but I could see from the expression of suffering on her face that things had gone wrong.

And then we were called in to the consultant, a woman in her thirties. Beside her sat a younger male colleague who seemed to be learning the ropes. The consultant gestured to us to sit down. She explained to her colleague that the client had come in and undergone emergency surgery, and that the baby had died.

"I'm sorry about what happened," she told Celeste.

I was still struggling to find the appropriate words to translate this when the consultant continued with her agenda. She explained the possible reasons for the problems that Celeste had had, and told Celeste that she wanted her to come in for investigation.

I translated this. Celeste was monosyllabic and uncommunicative. The consultant took out her Dictaphone. Ignoring us all, she dictated a couple of letters to colleagues requesting action. Then she gave Celeste detailed instructions of what to expect and how she was to respond. Did Celeste have any questions, she asked? Celeste said nothing.

"Quite honestly, I think she's still in shock at what you've just said!" I protested, but this drew no response from the consultant. The consultation took less than 5 minutes.

(*continued*)

Celeste looked a bit dazed, and I wasn't sure that she had retained the instructions that she had been given. I was also furious at the way that she had been treated. I motioned to her to wait while I got my time-sheet signed, then I patiently went through the instructions again. I was about to leave, when Celeste said "Would you do something for me?" "Yes of course!" I said.

Celeste then explained that they had taken a photograph of the dead baby, but at the time she didn't want to have anything to do with it. Now, she had changed her mind. They had told her that the photograph would be kept at the hospital. Could I help her to find it?

It didn't take long to locate the administrative section responsible for keeping these tragic records. Twenty minutes later, we were ushered into the office of a senior manager. She handed Celeste the photo of her dead baby.

Celeste's eyes filled up. She sat gazing at the photo, taking it in. The two of us were silent. After a pause, the manager remarked how upsetting it was when something like this happened. Did Celeste have anyone to talk to? I translated for her. Celeste shyly shook her head.

"Would she like to have someone to talk to?"

By the time we left, a referral for counseling had been made.

WHY USE AN INTERPRETER?

The use of an interpreter is both an equal opportunity and an access issue. It is good antidiscriminatory practice to use interpreters and translation services. People who are unable to access services because they are unable to communicate in English should be offered the use of an interpreter where necessary, and written information should be translated wherever possible. One woman told me that she hides the extent to which she is able to understand English in case she is told that she doesn't need an interpreter. Having access to an interpreter meant that she didn't need to struggle with the dual demands of listening and speaking in a different language, as well as taking on board medical information. It is also important to ask the client if he or she wants an interpreter, rather than make assumptions. They may also have a preference for an interpreter of a particular gender.

If your client is from a close-knit community, it is possible that he or she may know the translator, or know of the translator within the community. It is important to check this with the client and give him or her an opportunity to request translation services from someone not known to him or her or his or her extended family. Healthcare professionals need to check this sensitively and ensure that the client can reject a specific person without causing embarrassment.

If your client refuses a professional interpreter and comes with a nonprofessional to interpret (even if this is a family member or friend), it is important to make clear to the client that he or she can have a professional if he or she wants, and that you understand why he or she might prefer someone he or she knows. Genetic counseling sessions can cover very sensitive information, so it is important that the healthcare professional explains that to the client at the beginning of the consultation, so the client can appreciate the benefits of not relying on family members for translation. Family members or friends may not speak English adequately nor will they have had interpreting training. They won't have a professional framework of confidentiality and boundaries to guide them. They are unlikely to be truly impartial. They may have their own agenda about what they want to tell the client or share with the healthcare professional on behalf of the client. It can be a burden for the relative or friend to unwittingly learn of this sensitive information when he or she may have offered to translate simply to be helpful.

ASPECTS OF POWER

The use of a foreign-language interpreter complicates the process of communication. Three bridges are needed: between professional and client, professional and interpreter, and interpreter and client. Now there are three sets of trust to establish instead of one (for the sake of simplicity, I will assume one professional, one interpreter, and one client), and, in terms of social positioning, there is an added layer of differences of gender, class, race, and the like that can trigger potential collusion between any two of the three.

What effect does the use of an interpreter have on the balance of power between client and professional? The interpreter is booked by the professional and paid for by the professional's agency, but interpreters have their own professional code of neutrality to adhere to. Making sure that the client's voice is heard is seen as part of the professional role of interpreter. And interpreters have their own professional responsibility for responding appropriately to instances of racism and discrimination that may occur.

ISSUES OF TRUST

Trust is essential; yet when two people are involved in a conversation that the third is unable to understand, the third person is quick to feel excluded and suspicious. I think that professionals often find it hard to trust interpreters who are of the same ethnic origins as the clients. And it often seems to me that clients perceive interpreters and professionals who speak the same language and come from the same culture as being on the "same side."

Foreign-language interpreters stand at the intersection between professionals and clients of their services. At best, interpreters can be effective PR agents, helping clients to have confidence in professionals and the services they offer. This can be more difficult to achieve if professionals are uncomfortable, mistrustful, or uninformed about how to make effective use of an interpreter. And if the service that is being delivered by the professional is threadbare and contact with the client is poor, the position of the interpreter can be awkward. The interpreter has a responsibility for facilitating communication, but his or her control over the script is minimal.

In one particular case, I found myself in the strange situation of having to translate advice given by a health visitor that directly contradicted the views expressed by the midwife that I had translated the week before. They were giving advice on whether the new mother should ask her landlord to make her homeless. I know that professional opinions don't always agree, and yet I was surprisingly fazed by the situation. I came to the conclusion that I had unwittingly agreed with the first advice offered, then felt somewhat abashed by appearing to support the second source of advice. So much for neutrality!

In theory, an interpreter should translate word for word, relaying communication from one side of the bridge to another; in practice, this works only if both professional and interpreter are clear about their respective roles and confident about sticking to the boundaries of those roles. And word-for-word translation doesn't achieve the interpretation of meaning, which is something rather different (for example, a Tamil Asian had understandably but mistakenly filled in the costs of childcare as the cost of the child's food, diapers, and clothes.)

INTERPRETING FOR ASYLUM-SEEKERS AND REFUGEES

I encountered a further problem when interpreting for asylum-seekers and refugees: In many respects, they were treated the same as any other clients who came through the door, but this equitable treatment could result in inappropriate practice—whether through ignorance or a lack of imagination, it is difficult to say. I interpreted for a doctor who was baffled by a woman referring to having been in prison. The doctor had no concept of a regime that put women and children into detention camps to put pressure on their relatives—camps in which abuse was routine.

And it is worth remembering that asylum-seekers and refugees can also be people with mental illnesses, disabilities, and learning difficulties, or have their own idiosyncratic ways. I interpreted for one person who had a meandering short story approach to any answer and was in danger of being perceived as uncooperative because he was using the situation as a social encounter. Making an assessment through the medium of an interpreter has the potential for going badly wrong (see Box 12.3).

> **Box 12.3** Errors to Avoid when Using an Interpreter
>
> I have found that professionals often develop strange patterns of communication when they are faced with a client who doesn't understand what they say. They may begin to talk in disjointed phrases instead of sentences, rather as they would speak to a small child. I've done this myself, when I have been embarrassed in the face of noncomprehension. Yet it is much more difficult for the client to understand and much more difficult to translate. At the other extreme, long speeches that make several points put pressure on memory and make language harder to retrieve. Both clichés and jargon are difficult to translate from one language into another, and some expressions just don't translate.

Avoid the use of proverbs or slang as these are difficult to translate. I was stumped by the health visitor who said "He's a lovely child; enjoy him." It's a very English thing to say; there isn't a French equivalent. Through my head went the exhortations of waiters to enjoy your meal! "Mangez bien!" while the puzzled mother waited to hear what the health visitor had said.

Then there's the famous does-she-take-sugar-with-her-tea syndrome. (This is a reference to a famous radio show in the United Kingdom, written by disabled people for a disabled audience; it often challenges many misconceptions that non-disabled people have about disability.) The consultant turns to the interpreter and says: "Does she have any pain in the abdomen?" Obviously, the question should have been addressed directly to the client, not the interpreter. It's extraordinary how prevalent this way of behaving can be. I think that people are rendered uncomfortable or even distressed by the blank look of incomprehension that passes over someone's face, and they respond by defining the other person as stupid. This twisted form of communication goes hand in hand with a difficulty in looking the client in the eye. Yet the interaction is supposed to be between professional and client, not between the professional and the interpreter (see Box 12.4).

> **Box 12.4** Good Practice in Using Interpreters
>
> Best of all are those professionals who speak directly to their clients, using simple sentences, and maintaining eye contact as they do so. Then, if they keep their eyes on the client while the interpreter translates their words, they can note the client's non-verbal reactions to their words. In that way, they build up relationship and trust with the client, rather than with the interpreter. Ignore the interpreter if possible; health professionals need to have confidence that their words will be relayed accurately.

If you know a few words of the client's language, try them out. I think it must be music to the ears of those who wonder if anyone is going to be able to communicate with them.

Although the healthcare professional has responsibility for the clinical content of the appointment, it is worth bearing in mind that the translator may be a very useful source of information about the country the client is from, the culture, politics, geography, symbols and meaning relevant to the society or to particular ethnic groups. If the healthcare professional has a good understanding of these factors, it will only serve to enhance the communication with the client (Tribe & Thompson 2008).

In genetic consultations, it is hard to avoid medical jargon such as the terms "recessive inheritance," "gene," or "chromosome." The aim of the session is to make these terms clear to the client. It is advisable to review these words with the interpreter prior to the appointment, to check if there is a straightforward translation. If there isn't, it is advisable for the interpreter to use the English term and find ways to explain these words in their own language. The interpreter might find it useful to have some information on general genetic concepts, so that he or she can think of the best way to translate these complex ideas in advance.

The two case studies in Boxes 12.1 and 12.2 illustrate good practice and a session that leaves something to be desired.

The first case study shows how a professional who is both secure in his role and is confident about using an interpreter was able to offer a highly professional service. In the second case study, I believe that the visiting nurse was lacking in sensitivity and the consultant was embarrassed—first, by not being able to speak Celeste's language; second, by having to use an interpreter; and third, by the presence of a younger male colleague. I believe this led her to act inappropriately. The administrator saw Celeste as a human being and reacted as such.

SUMMARY

The necessity of using a foreign-language interpreter highlights issues of communication between professionals and the users of their services. I realize how great are the opportunities for misunderstanding between two people who apparently speak the same language; all of us need to be interpreters in our communication with others and wise to differences of culture and perspective.

Good Practice Guidelines: Making Effective Use of Interpreters

- Use a professional interpreter; try to match for age and gender when possible and avoid relying on family or friends. Never allow children to translate for their parents.

- Ask the client for what language he or she needs an interpreter, and try to book someone from the same country, who speaks the same dialect.
- Clinical responsibility rests with the healthcare professional. Have confidence in your professional role.
- Allow extra time for the consultation. Allow time in advance of the session to brief the interpreter about the purpose of the appointment, outline key genetic concepts, and enable him or her to brief you about any cultural issues. Allow time for translation, and allow time for a debriefing session with the interpreter.
- Be mindful of issues of confidentiality and trust when working with someone from a small language community (including the Deaf community) as the client may be anxious about being identifiable and mistrustful of an interpreter's professionalism.
- Create a good atmosphere in which each member of the triad feels able to ask for clarification if anything is unclear. Be respectful of your interpreter; he or she is an important member of the team who makes your work possible.
- Speak directly to and maintain eye contact with your client.
- Express yourself as you normally would.
- Use simple sentences; don't be tempted into short phrases.
- Recognize factors of race, gender, culture, age, and the like that might affect your communication.
- See also tips in Box 12.5.

Box 12.5 Good Practice in Communication with Clients

- Try to facilitate two-way traffic over the bridge.
- Use appropriate language; decode professional jargon.
- Be aware of professional power; work in a client-centered way.
- Recognize the effects of class, gender, race, age, culture, and the like on the communication process.
- Give clear information about your role and the service you offer, and check that this agenda is what the client was expecting.
- If using an interpreter, explain his or her role in the consultation to the client. (It is best to have negotiated this with the interpreter, prior to the appointment.)

RESOURCES

A guide to languages by country is available at http://www.ethnologue.com/country_index. asp (Accessed 9 April 2012)

The National Register of Public Service Interpreters (NRPSI) maintains a register of professional, qualified and accountable public service interpreters Available at http://www. nrpsi.co.uk/ (Accessed 9 April 2012)

REFERENCES

Tribe, R., & Thompson, K. (2008). *Working with interpreters in health settings: Guidelines for psychologists*. The British Psychological Society Professional Practice Board. Accessed April 8, 2012 from http://www.ucl.ac.uk/dclinpsy/training-handbook/chapters/handbook-pdf/appendix6

FURTHER READING

Cornwell , N. (2001). Piggy in the middle: Good practice and interpreters. In L. A. Cull and J. Roche (Eds.), *The law and social work: Contemporary issues for practice*. Basingstoke, UK: Palgrave.

13 Communication via the Telephone or Video Conferencing

Kelly Kohut and Kathryn Myhill

The more elaborate our means of communication the less we communicate.
—Joseph Priestley

Historically, genetic counseling in the United Kingdom has been delivered in a face-to-face hospital clinic setting. More recently, demands on genetic services, especially cancer genetic services have been changing. This has included an increase in referrals and more urgent referrals for genetic testing to aid in treatment planning, decision-making, and medical management. The cost of genetic testing will decrease dramatically in the next few years, and it will increasing become a mainstream service. An increase in the volume of clients using genetic services will dictate the development of innovative approaches to genetic counseling service delivery, for example, the use of a telephone clinic model.

Many genetic services may already use telephone consultations for a preclinic workup. Preliminary tests or investigations can be instigated as required. The genetic counselor can ensure relevant information, such as death certificates or pathology reports, is collated prior to a face-to-face appointment. If another relative is the ideal candidate for genetic testing, this can be explained over the telephone, which helps to both manage client expectations and avoid unnecessary hospital appointments. In the case of testing for cancer predisposition genes such as *BRCA1* and *BRCA2*, a symptomatic review of affected individuals can be undertaken, and candidates for fast-track testing can be identified to aid in surgical or treatment decision making.

Referrals are frequently received for individuals with family histories that do not meet criteria for genetic testing. They may be at moderately increased risk due to family history and need screening and lifestyle advice. They may have a risk similar to the population but be under the impression that their risk is much higher. These referrals could potentially be managed entirely by telephone and then discharged with a letter confirming appropriate surveillance recommendations. This allows prioritization of the face-to-face genetic counseling clinic for high-risk clients who are candidates for genetic testing and require more in-depth consultations about implications and clinical management options.

Clients may not understand why they have been referred and may be anxious about their appointment. A preclinic telephone assessment can be useful in outlining the purpose of the appointment and the potential benefits of genetic counseling and testing. This is useful in reducing nonattendance rates. This introduction is also useful in reducing client anxiety and managing expectations.

For those who are frail, immobile, struggling with the side effects of treatment, or living far away from the hospital, telephone consultation can provide a much more convenient, accessible service. It could reduce the need for additional hospital visits or a longer wait for an in-person consultation. For individuals with advanced disease with a personal or family history suspicious of a cancer genetic syndrome, basic family history details can be gleaned by phone and DNA storage arranged to help facilitate genetic assessment for children and other family members at a future point. This also obviates the need for an additional clinic visit when the client is fatigued and palliation of disease is the main focus.

Our own audit suggested satisfaction with telephone counseling and convenience of the service. This demonstrated the possibility for the telephone counseling model to provide a flexible, client-centered, and efficient service that could be adapted for other mainstream genetic services (Shanley et al. 2007).

The aim of this chapter is to offer practical advice on how to develop an effective telephone genetic counseling service. Suggestions will be provided regarding how to select suitable clients for the telephone clinic, literature to send to the client before the session, the family history questionnaire, methods of confirming diagnoses in the family, preparation for the telephone call, outline of a typical session, and how to address and overcome communication barriers. Case studies will be used to illustrate successes and challenges with telephone genetic counseling.

BACKGROUND

There are many types of clients for whom a telephone genetic counseling session may be appropriate. Some may be elderly, ill, or live a considerable distance from the hospital, which can make travel to a genetics center difficult and sometimes costly. Individuals who are working full-time may struggle to take time off work for a hospital appointment. For those at high risk of a genetic disorder, it may not always be possible to complete genetic counseling by telephone, although there is a place for this in some cases. Clients at lower risk may benefit from a review of their family history by telephone and reassurance that there is a low likelihood of a genetic predisposition in the family. Recommendations for screening may still be given, even if the family history does not meet criteria for genetic testing. Some clients would not pursue genetic counseling if a face-to-face visit was required but will participate in telephone counseling if this is offered (Sutphen et al. 2010). This may be for various reasons (e.g., fear of visiting the hospital following a traumatic illness in the family, which can back painful memories and sometimes cause a person to avoid hospitals unless an absolute emergency occurs). A client may feel that, as a healthy person, it is unnecessarily anxiety-provoking to go to a hospital appointment, and this may result in avoidance of facing his or her genetic risk.

In the case of cancer susceptibility syndromes, clients are sometimes referred soon after a diagnosis of cancer to investigate the possibility of genetic testing to aid in treatment or surgical decision making. This is becoming a more common practice as the potential for targeted therapy continues to be explored (Fong et al. 2009), and client acceptance of treatment-focused genetic testing has been high (Meiser et al. 2012). Several research studies have been completed suggesting that disclosure of BRCA1/BRCA2 genetic test results by telephone does not significantly affect knowledge gained (Helmes, Culver, & Bowen 2006), outcome (Doughty Rice et al. 2010), or satisfaction, particularly when given a choice up front about whether to receive results by telephone or face-to-face (Baumanis et al. 2009).

Clinical judgment must be used to identify situations in which telephone genetic counseling, particularly for disclosure of test results, is not appropriate. Further study is needed in this area, and a set of guidelines would be valuable to genetic counselors. One experienced genetic team has developed a protocol for testing for Huntington disease in which telephone counseling by a psychologist is used initially to explore a client's motivations for pursuing testing. However, results are never disclosed by telephone, even when requested by the client, due to the sensitive nature of the information and the potential for psychological distress (Dufrasne et al. 2011). BRCA1/BRCA2 genetic test results are often disclosed by telephone by genetic counselors, although many have encountered situations in which they felt this method of disclosure was not ideal (Bradbury et al. 2011). A list of possible pros and cons of telephone counseling is presented in Table 13.1.

PREPARING FOR THE CONSULTATION

Selecting Clients for the Telephone Clinic

Client characteristics are often used by genetic counselors in deciding when to offer genetic counseling by telephone, such as the likelihood of a positive genetic test result, strength of the family history, or personal history of cancer. However, it is not clear that these factors have significantly impacted the method of results disclosure and further research is needed, including prospective studies (Doughty Rice

Table 13.1 Potential advantages and disadvantages of genetic counseling by telephone

Advantages	Disadvantages
1. Wider access to genetic specialists	1. External distractions and lack of privacy if client does not have a quiet place to speak
2. Convenience for the client (less time off work, less time and expense for travel)	
3. Improved accessibility to genetics service for client living a long distance from the genetics center	2. Lack of nonverbal communication
	3. Loss or reduction of reimbursement to genetics center
4. Potential to decrease waiting time for the appointment	4. Decreased opportunity for rapport-building between healthcare provider and client
5. Facilitation of rapid genetic test results to aid decision-making for treatment/surgery or entry into clinical trials	5. Client may not grasp importance of genetic counseling when sent an appointment for telephone consultation
6. Facilitation of DNA storage/genetic assessment for other family members	

et al. 2011). A suggested list of features to consider when deciding whether telephone counseling is appropriate is presented in Table 13.2.

The Clinic Booking Process

If there is an option of telephone clinic or face-to-face clinic for new clients (initial consultations), referrals should be triaged by a senior member of staff to assess suitability for telephone counseling. If the client has been seen at another hospital previously, it is useful to request copies of relevant histopathology reports or mutation reports in advance of the appointment. Members of a family in which a gene mutation has already been identified might benefit from an introductory telephone session to prepare them for further in-depth discussion at the face-to-face clinic. Additional considerations are outlined in Table 13.2.

Preparing for the Consultation

A family history questionnaire can be sent to the client upon receipt of the referral letter, with the aim of creating a pedigree prior to the first appointment. This is central to an adequate precounseling assessment of risk and testing options in the family. It is useful to include a leaflet about the telephone genetic counseling clinic with the client's appointment letter. This should explain that, following the telephone consultation, it might be necessary to arrange a subsequent appointment in person; it is best to prepare clients for this possibility in advance to avoid unrealistic expectations of necessarily managing the whole genetic counseling process by telephone.

Table 13.2 Personal client characteristics to take into account when deciding whether telephone genetic counseling is an appropriate option.

Client Characteristics	Considerations
Personal history of cancer or serious illness	(+) Clients who are elderly, frail, in ill health, or receiving frequent and debilitating treatment for their disease may already have a full schedule of medical appointments and might value the flexibility of genetic counseling by telephone.
	(+) Individuals who are unwell due to metastatic cancer or another serious condition may need to be seen quickly, if not for genetic testing then perhaps to discuss the option of DNA storage. This would allow for future referral of family members to discuss taking genetic testing forward on the stored sample.
	(+) Client might be candidate for clinical trial, targeted treatment, or risk-reducing surgery if rapid genetic testing is performed and a mutation is identified.
	(−) Complicated or highly emotionally charged discussion may be difficult by telephone.
Likelihood of positive genetic test result	(+) Client has known about a mutation in the family for some time, is expecting to be positive, and has given options a lot of thought already.
	(+) There is a very low likelihood of a positive result, and client needs reassurance counseling and to be told that genetic testing is unlikely to be helpful.
	(−) There is a high likelihood of a positive result but the client does not know anything about the genetic condition yet or has difficulties with language or comprehension.
Personal implications of a positive result	(+) Client has already been treated for a disease and/or taken risk-reducing measures and is considering genetic testing mainly to provide information to family members.
	(−) Client has all of the genetic risk ahead of her and many implications to consider if positive (e.g., a young woman who has not yet had children learning she has a BRCA gene mutation).
Mental health	(+) Client has no history of mental health issues.
	(−) Client has a history of mental health issues and problems with coping strategies. Might need additional supportive counseling, referral to psychologist
Support system	(+) Client has a strong network of family/friends.
	(−) Client is lacking social support and is more likely to require additional counseling.

(continued)

Table 13.2 (Continued)

Client Characteristics	Considerations
Education and understanding	(+) Client has a previous understanding or easily grasps genetic concepts and the implications to self and family.
	(−) If it is apparent from the referral letter or initial telephone consultation that information is not well understood, consider further in-person counseling.

Considerations for each characteristic are presented with a plus sign (+) or minus sign (−) indicating a positive or negative indication for using the telephone clinic model.

Planning for Counseling by Telephone

A letter notifying the client of the planned telephone consultation should be sent to maximize the likelihood that the client will find a suitable location for a private conversation and be ready to accept the incoming call. If this is sent far in advance of the appointment, a reminder letter will help to ensure that the client is still expecting the call. It is preferable to give a timeframe when the person may be called, for example between 9 a.m. and 12 p.m. or between 1 p.m. and 5 p.m., rather than committing to a specific time slot. This will give flexibility for attempts to reach other clients scheduled for that clinic if the first person does not answer right away. Some telephone companies offer a free screening service for nuisance calls; however, this service will also block any unidentified number. Most outgoing calls from hospitals will present as a blocked number, making it impossible to get through to the client. It is helpful to include some variation of the following in the appointment letter: "Please be advised that the switchboard automatically withholds our telephone number to ensure client confidentiality. If the telephone number detailed above does not accept this type of incoming call, please ensure you advise us of a suitable alternative number to call you on." It is good practice to include spaces for clients to provide multiple telephone numbers (including a mobile number if available) on the family history questionnaire.

A checklist for items to include in the appointment letter is as follows:

- Date of appointment
- Time to be called (e.g., use a timespan of 3–4 hours for a clinic of three clients) and likely length of call
- Telephone number(s) to be contacted on, and request for client to call the genetics service to add alternative number(s) if necessary
- Anticipated length of the call
- Assurance that confidentiality will be maintained
- Note about call blocking services not accepting calls from the hospital
- Contact details for the genetics service

Communication Challenges

Genetic counseling by telephone presents several unique challenges. Unlike the traditional hospital-based clinic appointment, the client may not have access to a quiet, private location. Due to full-time employment or other commitments that prevent being at home during working hours, the client might need to be called on a mobile telephone. When telephoning, it is useful to keep in mind that confidentiality is important and expected, even if a client has provided a work or mobile number. It is best to ensure the client is indeed the person on the other end of the line before disclosing the purpose of the call. If someone else answers, it is preferable to state that it is a personal call and ask when the client is likely to be available. If pressed for more information, the genetic counselor can politely state the need, to discuss the purpose of the call directly with the person involved.

Reaching clients by telephone can be difficult, even when an appointment letter is sent in advance. The genetic counselor may wish to avoid leaving a voicemail message due to concerns about confidentiality, but in practice this would make it very difficult to complete all of the scheduled calls in the time allotted for clinic. Messages can be left as long as they are suitably vague so that if another person listens to the message, the purpose of the call will not be immediately obvious. It may be sufficient to leave the genetic counselor's name and telephone number asking the client to call back at a suitable time and noting that another call will be attempted later that morning/afternoon. If a second message is necessary, it is worthwhile stating that a telephone call had been scheduled for that day, in case the client did not recognize that the first message was from the genetics service. It is suggested that the following statement or something similar be included in the new appointment letter sent to clients whom the genetic counselor is unable to reach: "As part of the NHS Guidelines relating to Information Governance concerning client confidentiality, our telephone number is automatically withheld and we are not able to leave detailed messages on answering machines."

Once connected, it is wise to check that it is a suitable time for the client to have a discussion about genetics, even though the appointment was prearranged. This emphasizes that the genetic counselor is providing the client with undivided attention and aiming to get the same in return. As with in-person genetic counseling sessions, contracting is a key part of the telephone consultation. The client may think it unusual to have a medical appointment by telephone, and it is useful to explain the purpose of the telephone clinic and the possibility of future in-person or telephone appointments, as appropriate. The genetic counselor should stop to check that the purpose of the appointment has been understood and to ask whether there is anything else the client wishes to discuss. Current medical symptoms should be assessed. If there are significant concerns, these symptoms should be discussed with the geneticist and the client called back for further instruction. It can be very helpful to explore the client's motivations for pursuing genetic counseling, as well as his or her expectations. Some may not be fully aware of why they were referred, particularly when referred by the general practitioner.

Distractions

Often, clients do wish to have genetic counseling and have genuine concerns to discuss, but find themselves in an awkward position when the telephone call is received. They may be caring for small children who need their attention, at a workplace where there is little privacy, or out doing shopping or other tasks while on their mobile phone. The genetic counselor should ensure that the client is in the best possible place to receive the call and explain that it is necessary to find a time to speak when full attention can be given. If the client is at work, it may be possible to go into a private meeting room and receive a call back on a landline telephone. If the client is about to go out to drop off children at school, it might be better to arrange a suitable time to speak later in the day. One of the disadvantages of the telephone clinic is difficulty finding an ideal time to speak. This can significantly add to the time needed for the clinic and can be frustrating for the genetic counselor; however, if the client appreciates the importance of the information to be discussed, it should be possible to come to an agreement. Trying to perform a genetic counseling session by telephone when the client is constantly interrupted and cannot concentrate is unlikely to be beneficial to either party.

Language Barriers

Sometimes, it is not evident from the referral letter that the client's first language is not English. Even if the client speaks English at a reasonably proficient level, it may be preferable to offer an interpreter to ensure that the complicated nature of the discussion will be adequately understood. With advance notice, the genetic counselor can arrange to use a telephone language line service for translation; however, for particularly complex cases, it would be better to change the appointment to face-to-face and arrange for an interpreter to be present. This allows for better flow of dialogue and the addition of body language cues to gauge how the information is received. If the client opts to have the consultation by telephone, additional time must be allowed for translation. Generally, the consultation should be expected to take at least twice as long, and clinic scheduling will need to be adjusted accordingly.

Taking a Family History

Ideally, the family history will have been collected via a questionnaire and a pedigree constructed prior to the appointment. This will save time in the session because it can be a protracted and frustrating process to get clients to accurately explain how relatives are related without the aid of a printed family tree. It is useful to confirm that the family history from the questionnaire is correct when speaking with a client by telephone. This is also a way to break the ice, build rapport, and set the scene for the genetic risk assessment; unfortunately, this relies solely on verbal communication. If the family history is very complicated, for example involving multiple partners, consanguinity, or uncertainties about how individuals are related, it might be appropriate to arrange a follow-up visit in the clinic for further clarification. In the time between the telephone consultation and the clinic appointment, the genetic counselor can arrange to confirm information about the family. For example, death certificates can be requested online by the client through the General Register Office; this can be helpful to confirm or clarify a diagnosis, which is critical to the overall risk assessment. For cancer diagnoses, there is a network of Cancer Registries around the United Kingdom. Information requests can be sent to confirm the type of cancer with which relatives were diagnosed. If the person is alive, a signed consent form is required. With a consent form, the genetic counselor could also try writing to the hospital where the person was treated.

Dealing with Anxious Clients

People who are referred for genetic counseling have usually been diagnosed with a condition themselves or experienced it in their family. In many cases, there is some level of anxiety surrounding the possibility of a genetic predisposition being passed on in the family. If meeting clients in person, this is easier to detect by taking account of facial expression and body language. In the telephone clinic, attention must be paid to more subtle clues. Tone of voice and pace of speech is important. It may be difficult to slow down highly distressed clients and keep them focused on the genetic counseling agenda. They may become highly emotive when discussing the personal or family history of a disease. Silence can be useful in face-to-face appointments to allow time for clients to process and express their emotions. In telephone consultations, silence can cause misunderstandings, and it is crucial to let the client know that the genetic counselor is still there and is highly attentive. Affirming phrases such as "Yes," "I see," and "Go on" are useful to keep the conversation flowing. The genetic counselor should use a calm, clear voice and a slow pace to encourage the client to share information and to promote a relaxed and open atmosphere for discussion. Checking how the information is received along the way or at the end of the consultation can be helped with a phrase such as "Has any of this information been surprising to hear today?" Offering a subsequent in-person appointment within a short timeframe could be helpful for certain clients who are emotionally fragile and feel there is too much information to absorb via a telephone conversation. There is also an opportunity for the genetic counselor to recognize limitations; for those clients who have deep-seated psychological problems that are not solely linked to the genetic problem, a referral to psychological support service may be appropriate.

Visual Aids

The written summary letter is a vital tool to reinforce the information discussed during a telephone counseling session. If there are concerns about communication with a visual learner, it can be helpful to include aids such as a copy of the pedigree, leaflets, or links to websites for information and sources of support. It is useful to perform frequent checks during the consultation to ensure the information is being understood. For those clients whose learning style is more visual, it may be worthwhile considering a video conference (Zilliacus et al. 2010) rather than a simple telephone call, if resources permit (see Boxes 13.1 and 13.2).

Box 13.1 Case Study 1

Sarah was referred by her general practitioner (GP) for risk assessment and screening advice regarding her family history of bowel cancer. Although there was a history of bowel cancer in the family, Sarah's focus was on the recent loss of her sister to pancreatic cancer and whether this increased her own risk of pancreatic cancer. The family history included other cancers, and a cluster of breast cancer in paternal relatives. Genetic assessment included consideration of bowel cancer risk and possible Lynch syndrome as well as possible *BRCA* testing in a relative affected by breast cancer. However, it was evident that the best starting point for the first telephone consultation was rapport building, to explore Sarah's perception of cancer risks due to family history and to address some of the feelings surrounding the loss of her sister that were influencing her risk perception. It was important to take the time to outline that, on the whole, cancer is a sporadic disease, rather than a strongly inherited trait and to explain how screening of the pancreas was still being evaluated in the research setting. As there was potentially a lot of information to digest, a plan was agreed to arrange a baseline colonoscopy and mammogram and to break down genetic assessment into two parts. A consent form was sent out for Sarah's niece to consent to tissue block testing of their mother's pancreatic tumour tissue (immunohistochemistry testing to assess for Lynch syndrome). Once the testing was initiated, a clinic appointment would then be made a few weeks later to meet Sarah face-to-face to discuss the results and to decide on ongoing bowel screening recommendations. At that point, the place of *BRCA* testing could be further discussed.

The initial telephone appointment was useful for both Sarah and the genetics service. The genetic counselor was able to identify that Sarah's main issue was not the same as the reason why she was referred and was able to both acknowledge her issues around her bereavement and her concern of pancreatic cancer and manage her expectations of the genetics service. Information was obtained so that initial testing could be undertaken prior to a face-to-face appointment, so that the risk assessment would be more accurate. As the risk assessment could prove to be complicated, the initial appointment gave Sarah enough information to answer her immediate questions and was a foundation to build upon in subsequent appointments.

Box 13.2 Case Study 2

Two identical twin sisters, Ann and Tina (unaffected), aged 35, and another sister, Ruth, aged 42 (affected with breast cancer) were referred individually for genetic testing after a *BRCA* mutation was identified in another sister, Fiona. Fiona was 38 and affected by metastatic breast cancer. We spoke to all three sisters about genetic testing separately in the telephone clinic; this revealed different individual issues and perspectives regarding genetic testing and highlighted some family issues. Fiona's poor prognosis had a significant emotional impact on all three sisters and the family as a whole. The identical twin sisters Ann and Tina had different agendas regarding genetic testing; Ann was very keen to pursue predictive testing, whereas Tina was more ambivalent about finding out if she had the mutation and coping with that knowledge. Tina was also separately dealing with some difficult relationship issues. In both Ann and Tina's consultations, we outlined the fact that a test result for one twin would likely be the same for the other and therefore both sisters needed to be in the right place to take forward predictive testing.

Ruth wanted to have genetic testing to confirm that she had inherited the *BRCA* mutation and so that her teenage children could consider predictive testing at a future point. As Ruth was over 40, a confirmatory test would also clarify her ovarian cancer risk, and prophylactic oophorectomy could be a consideration. Ruth was keen to consider this procedure, and some of the implications of this surgery were discussed in the telephone consultation. Ruth was aware that both Ann and Tina were considering predictive testing, but acknowledged her anxiety about them having to deal with a positive test result. However, the consultation gave the opportunity to discuss the possible positive aspects of finding out carrier status, such as making decisions about risk-reducing surgery and exploring the need to make an autonomous decision.

Speaking to all three sisters separately gave us the opportunity to explore their individual perspectives, understandings, and feelings surrounding genetic testing and to do some crucial groundwork in exploring the implications specific to their situation. It gave Ann and Tina time to pause and consider each other's needs and the importance of timing when considering taking predictive testing forward. We were able to address some of Ruth's anxieties regarding testing in her sisters and facilitate confirmatory testing by mail following this.

SUMMARY

In summary, the telephone genetic counseling clinic can be a useful tool to reach clients who are at low risk of a genetic condition; live far away from the genetics center; find it difficult to travel due to illness, cost, or frailty; are able to understand and assimilate genetic risk information easily; or need a rapid genetic test (by post) to aid in treatment planning. Telephone genetic counseling has been found to be comparable to the traditional model in outcome and client satisfaction. The telephone clinic model can provide flexibility and convenience for the client and the counselor, but many times a follow-up in-person appointment will be beneficial. Telephone counseling is not appropriate for all clients, and it would be prudent to consider prior psychological history and the complexity of the case when triaging referrals into the telephone or face-to-face clinic.

Recommendations for practice and practical tips include:

- Carefully select clients for the telephone clinic.
- Be mindful of scheduling.
- Prepare for the telephone call.
- Provide pre-and post-consultation documentation.
- Be sensitive to situations in which a telephone consultation is not ideal.
- Explore solutions to language and communication barriers.

Ideally, genetic services will have access to both telephone and face-to-face clinics to meet the growing needs of the population being served. Demands on genetic services are increasing, and the telephone clinic model is one component to consider in planning innovative solutions.

REFERENCES

Baumanis, L., Evans, J. P., Callanan, N., & Susswein, L. R. (2009). Telephoned BRCA1/2 genetic test results: Prevalence, practice and patient satisfaction. *Journal of Genetic Counseling, 18,* 447–463.

Bradbury, A. R., Patrick-Miller, L., Fetzer, D., Egleston, B., Cummings, S. A., Forman, A., et al. (2011). Genetic counselors opinions of, and experience with telephone communication of BRCA1/2 test results. *Clinical Genetics, 79,* 125–131.

Doughty Rice, C., Ruschman, J.G., Martin, L. J., Manders, J. B., & Miller, E. (2010). Retrospective comparison of patient outcomes after in-person and telephone results disclosure counseling for BRCA1/2 genetic testing. *Familial Cancer, 9,* 203–212.

Dufrasne, S., Roy, M., Galvez, M., & Rosenblatt, D. S. (2011). Experience over fifteen years with a protocol for predictive testing for Huntington disease. *Molecular Genetics and Metabolism, 102,* 494–504.

Fong, P. C., Boss, D. S., Yap, T. A., Tutt, A., Wu, P., Mergui-Roelvink, M., et al. (2009). Inhibition of poly(ADP-ribose) polymerase in tumors from BRCA mutation carriers. *New England Journal of Medicine, 361,*123–134.

Helmes, A. W., Culver, J. O., & Bowen, D. J . (2006). Results of a randomized study of telephone versus in-person breast cancer risk counseling. *Patient Education and Counseling, 64,* 96–103.

Meiser, B., Gleeson, M., Kasparian, N., Barlow-Stewart, K., Ryan, M., Watts, K., et al. (2012). There is no decision to make: Experiences and attitudes toward treatment-focused genetic testing among women diagnosed with ovarian cancer. *Gynecological Oncology, 124,*153–157.

Shanley, S., Myhill, K., Doherty, R., Arden-Jones, A., Hall, S., Vince, C. et al. (2007). Delivery of cancer genetics services: The Royal Marsden telephone clinic model. *Familial Cancer, 6*, 213–219.

Sutphen, R., Davila, B., Shappell, H., Holtje, T., Vadaparampil, S., Friedman, S., et al. (2010). Real world experience with cancer genetic counselling via telephone. *Familial Cancer, 9*, 681–689.

Zilliacus, E. M., Meiser, B., Lobb, E. A., Kirk, J., Warwick, L., & Tucker, K. (2010). Women's experience of telehealth cancer genetic counseling. *Journal of Genetic Counseling, 19*, 463–472.

Index